A Feather in My Wig

A Feather in My Wig

OVARIAN CANCER: CURED

Twelve~~ ~~Years and Going Strong!
Seventeen

by

Barbara R. Van Billiard

Foreword by
Theodore C. Barton, M.D., FACS

PETER E. RANDALL PUBLISHER
PORTSMOUTH, NEW HAMPSHIRE
2005

Cover design: Nancy Landroche

Peter E. Randall Publisher
Box 4726
Portsmouth, NH 03802-4726

Distributed by University Press of New England
Hanover and London

Library of Congress Cataloging-in-Publication Data

Van Billiard, Barbara, 1929
    A feather in my wig : ovarian cancer cured: twelve years and
going strong! / by Barbara R. Van Billiard; foreword by
Theodore C. Barton.
        p. cm .
    ISBN 0-914339-69-9 (alk. paper)
    1. Van Billiard, Barbara, 1929—-Health. 2. Ovaries—Cancer-
-Patients—United States—Biography. I. Title.
RC280.08V36 1998
362.1'9699465'0092—dc2l
[b]

                                            98-46047
                                               CIP

For

Russ

and

Theodore C. Barton, M.D.

My Grandma

My Grandma had ovarian cancer. Ovarian cancer is one of the worst types of cancer because it is hard to diagnose. Usually by the time that the cancer is found, it is too late to be successfully treated. Hardly any people survive. Most people who have ovarian cancer die from it, but luckily my Grandma didn't. She does not intend to get her cancer back. My Grandma had surgery and then chemotherapy treatment for seven months, which made her lose her hair and get really sick.

At first, my Grandma had an immediate thought of death, but then quickly said that she was going to live and beat that cancer. My Grandma prayed a lot because she wanted to keep herself alive. My Grandma did imagery which means to visualize good things that you want to happen to you. My Grandma thought of a big thing going through her body and erasing all of the cancer cells away and everything would be gone.

Everyone who knows my Grandma thinks that it is a miracle that she lived. My Grandma got a lot of love and support. She says God helped her by giving her that miracle to keep her alive. Her family and friends helped her through everything. There were different churches with different religions that were praying for my Grandma. My Grandma's doctor, Dr. Barton, helped her and kept her alive and now is a family friend. My Grandma used self healing tapes and books also. As soon as my Grandma was strong enough, she exercised daily. She jogs five miles a day, cross country skis in the winter, and rides her bike around the block. Because of doing all of these things my Grandma got better.

After eight, long, tough, painful years of cancer, my Grandma lost her cancer. She lost it because of the surgery she had by one of the best surgeons in the world, the other operations, and love, support, and all of the wonderful miracles. She kept trying to get better and she did. She met her goal and everyone was proud of her for that. With all of the surgery, it left her with some health problems and she had to limit some activities. One of her greatest accomplishments is in doing lots of helping with cancer patients and showing them how to use imagery.

My Grandma is doing well and is the strongest person that I know. She deals with things well. As you can see, my Grandma has overcome lots of different things. A lot of cancer patients give up faith and lose hope, unlike my Grandma who is the complete opposite of that and would never do that.

Another thing that is great about my Grandma is that she not only helps herself, she helps others too. She helps cancer patients and tells them to have faith and they will feel and get better. When she was a nurse she would tell them to be strong and to have faith too. She also taught them imagery.

My Grandma has a loving heart, helpfulness inside, and lots of faith. She has always been there for me and I will always be there for her because I love her very much. I am proud to have a Grandma who is alive to this day.

Lindsay Landroche, age 10
Civic Oration Presentation
Berwick, Maine, Elementary School
February 1994

Contents

Acknowledgments

My heartfelt thanks to my daughter
Nancy Landroche, who finally discovered
how I knew where the four-leaf clovers grow.

Aware of my computer illiteracy, Nancy
lovingly gave of her valuable time and her
boundless talents to make my story a reality.

My loving gratitude to Nancy Bray, who was
and is always there for me and my family.

My sincere thanks to Ruth Dow for reading
the manuscript. Her thoughtful
suggestions were an enormous help.

I am most grateful to Dr. Richard T. Penson for his
assistance in updating the Second printing.

Foreword

Barbara Van Billiard performs a great service to women in writing the story of her successful battle with that great nemesis, ovarian cancer. No other cancer of the female reproductive system carries such grim survival statistics. As you read of her fight, you will experience first hand an account of the rigors she endured, the mental discipline she brought to bear—a discipline that ensured survival.

Barbara Van Billiard is a medically sophisticated registered nurse, a graduate of the New England Baptist Hospital School of Nursing and the University of New Hampshire. In spite of her medical background, ovarian cancer progressed to an advanced stage before the tumor was recognized. This is almost invariably the case. The tumor arises in the ovary and most often spreads through the abdominal cavity before discovery. The cold statistics project approximately a 30 percent five year survival.

Discouraging news for any patient but, when looked at closely, these statistics should convey the information that there are those who will engage this adversary and live. Survival requires aggressive surgery, followed by chemotherapy, and all this coupled with an indomitable determination to live. Barbara's account of all these signal events are accurate and may be believed.

Going beyond the insults of surgery and chemotherapy, a necessary element is that the patient inwardly project the imagery of survival. Barbara expertly describes the mobilization of those powerful forces, forces that transcend the skill of the surgeon. These mechanisms mobilize the endorphins and cytokines that implement and enhance the immune response directed to the destruction of the invading cancer.

Barbara Van Billiard is a cancer survivor. The message in this volume will go out providing assurance that this disease need not be fatal.

Theodore C. Barton, M.D., FACS
Chief, Department of Gynecology
New England Baptist Hospital
Assistant Clinical Professor of Surgery
Harvard Medical School

Prologue

At the time of my diagnosis of ovarian cancer and during my treatment, I knew no survivors of this life-threatening disease who could reach out to me and say, "Look, here I am—I fought hard to survive and you can too!"

What I had were the depressing memories of patients whom I had cared for during my nursing career before the days of chemotherapy. Women diagnosed with ovarian cancer had very little chance of survival. Through the years, the very words "ovarian cancer" struck terror in my heart.

My personal nightmare began in 1986 when I became a victim of the "silent killer."

People who know what I have experienced and survived besiege me with questions. What were my symptoms? How did I know where to go? Who was my surgeon? How was I diagnosed? How was I treated? I can feel the fear being expressed that all of these women are living with the horrible reality that they might become victims of this insidious disease and not be aware of it until too late.

Now, twelve years later, with no recurrence of cancer, I feel obligated to answer these questions, to explain some of my survival techniques, and especially to offer hope.

Writing about my illness was not undertaken without fear and reluctance. Much of what I had endured since 1986 was painful and embittering, and the idea of reliving these incidents through literary exposure caused overwhelming ambivalence.

Dr. Deepak Chopra, in his book *Ageless Body, Timeless Mind*, authenticates my fears: "A remembered stress which is only a wisp of thought," he writes, "releases the same flood of destructive hormones as the stress itself."

Believing that as a long-term survivor I had a commitment to share my triumph, I realized I would never have peace of mind or of soul until I wrote this book as a form of HOPE—the embodiment of survival. I am convinced that the chances of surviving cancer are greatly increased by having a passionate desire to live—a raging, fighting spirit, and HOPE!

While putting up a good fight is essential, it is important to remember that, as in all battles, there are times when we need to ask for help, to realize that it is okay to stop for a breather and regroup before we can effectually proceed to win the war. Hope, however, must stay constant; it can't stop and rest.

The poet Emily Dickinson wrote:

> Hope is the thing with feathers
> that perches in the soul
> and sings the tune without the words
> and never stops at all.

Locke and Colligan, in *The Healer Within*, explaining coping strategies used by survivors of the Nazi death camps, tell how psychiatrist Joel Densdale, through interviews to determine what kept them alive, found that the one attitude that surpassed all others was the human quality of "blind naked hope." Studies in this same book support that "hope has profound immunological effects."

The well-known prayer of Saint Francis includes the

line in which he implores that where there is despair, let there be hope. This book is my attempt to bring hope where there is despair, to let other women know that when the diagnosis is ovarian cancer, they must fight, hope, and survive. I did!

This account of my survival does not always flow along in a smooth, orderly sequence, as was typical of my life during these years.

Disclosure:
A Year of Fears

Misdiagnosed

In April 1985, I visited my gynecologist, Dr. A., in Boston. I had been his patient for about seven years, seeing him routinely every six months. During this visit I told him that I had experienced some vaginal spotting unrelated to my estrogen replacement therapy cycle. He performed an endometrial biopsy in the office. The results were negative. I sometimes wonder if this could have been the first symptom, as some ovarian cancers secrete a hormone that causes bleeding.

In October 1985 I returned to Dr. A. for another routine examination. He discovered a large pelvic mass, which he believed was probably a large fibroid, but felt he could not take the chance that it could be ovarian cancer. So that very day, he sent me to a hospital in the Boston area to a radiologist who, I was told, was outstanding in the field of ultrasonography.

I had a sonogram of my pelvic area, which I observed on the screen, and it did show, according to the radiologist, a large uterine fibroid with a normal left ovary and the right ovary not visualized. To quote him, this means "the ovary is small, so it wouldn't push through the intestines and gas and so forth . . . so we just don't worry when we don't see it."

I took his word for it and the next day I talked with Dr.

A. on the phone. He agreed with the diagnosis and that what we should do was have a repeat ultrasound in three months. I was delighted that the mass was not ovarian and would not require a hysterectomy, with the holidays forthcoming. I felt quite comfortable with this diagnosis.

The summer and fall of 1985 had been a happy and healthy time for me (so I thought)—my stamina allowed me to be running about seven miles each day. Apparently this amount of pounding the pavement was too much for me because I developed ischeal bursitis, an inflammation of one of the lower pelvic bones, and pulled right hamstring muscles. This coincided with the discovery of my so-called large uterine fibroid. I had daily physical therapy and stopped all exercise. During this time I felt a pulling sensation and discomfort in my right groin. I casually mentioned it to my orthopedist, whom I had told of my upcoming surgery for a large fibroid and he reassured me that it was no doubt related to that problem and to mention it to my gynecologist. I have little doubt that this was a symptom of my enlarged right ovary.

A few weeks later I returned for another pelvic exam, which, after having a Fleet enema, would provide more accuracy in determining my diagnosis. Again, I was told that I had a large uterine fibroid. In three weeks, I was to have my second ultrasound at the same small hospital in Brookline.

This ultrasound was scheduled for the 10th of January 1986. One of the preparations for this test is to drink large amounts of fluid. Before I left home I had juice, two cups of coffee, and took a container of water with me in the car.

Russ, my husband of then thirty-three years, drove while I drank water during this sixty-mile ride. Halfway to Boston, I realized that the copious amounts of liquid had not gone beyond my stomach. As we entered Storrow Drive, I felt horribly nauseated and up came torrents of liquid in the form of projectile vomiting. Needless to say, the car was inundated, and I was pretty well covered. Somehow Russ escaped the mess and remained calm enough to fight his way through the Boston traffic on a most harrowing trip to the hospital.

Of course, the ultrasound was canceled, and we made a hurried trip to the office of my gynecologist, where I continued vomiting. There was little doubt that I had an intestinal obstruction, so I was admitted to the New England Baptist Hospital (NEBH) where I spent the weekend.

The obstruction, which was in the small intestine, somehow cleared without intervention. During this hospitalization my gynecologist consulted with a surgeon. The conclusion seemed to be that my problem was the result of pressure from the fibroid or possibly from a long-standing ventral hernia. These two physicians decided that I required no emergency surgery but should have a hysterectomy early in February, after my husband's retirement. In the meantime, I would have my second ultrasound, but instead of another trip to Boston, I would have it in a hospital nearer home.

I know my guardian angel was with me that weekend and I have thanked God over and over that no emergency surgery was performed, for I doubt I would have been a "survivor." Although I didn't realize it, I was not in the best physical condition and, even more significant, I would not have had the surgical expertise of Dr. Theodore Barton, to whom I owe my life.

On the 16th of January in 1986 I went to a nearby hospital for my second ultrasound. I noticed on the radiology requisite that it was "to rule out cholelithiasis [gallstones] and ovarian enlargement." I again watched the procedure on the screen and read the negative report, which stated that both left and right ovaries are visualized and do not appear enlarged. This report was sent to my physician in Boston. Meanwhile, I was becoming extremely uncomfortable with a lot of pressure on my bladder and bowel, and my abdomen began to swell. But I thought, "Well, I've had two negative ultrasounds . . ." I looked like a typical ovarian cancer patient and I had seen many before, but I just knew that I didn't have it. I had had "two negative ultrasounds!" Ignorance may be bliss, but in this case it almost killed me.

I gave two pints of blood autologously (that is, my own blood, if I required transfusions), for use during surgery and was admitted to the New England Baptist Hospital on the 5th of February 1986. I looked as if I were in my sixth month of pregnancy. I was scheduled to have a hysterectomy the next day. Shortly after I was admitted, I was walking in the hall to be weighed when an old friend and surgeon, Dr. Kenneth Warren, with whom I had worked as a student and greatly respected, walked by. I hadn't seen him in years and welcomed a chat. He looked at me and said, "Oh, ovarian . . . hmm?" I said, "Oh no—just a fibroid."

The "A Team"

I still don't know if that encounter with Dr. Warren had anything to do with what transpired or if it was due to the intervention of an observant nurse. A short time later a gentleman walked into my room, pulled up a chair, and introduced himself as Dr. Theodore Barton, who was going to take over my case. This is the man who would save my life and become a very special friend to me and to my family.

He said, "You may not like me very well because I've got to do dreadful things to you. We've got to build you up and give you back your two pints of blood immediately, put a nasogastric tube into your stomach, do a surgical cut down so we can do some hyperalimentation and give you fluids, and postpone your surgery until the 10th of February." Feeling comfortable about being in Dr. Barton's care, I told him to proceed with whatever needed to be done.

Later that day, Dr. Barton's oncology nurse, Nancy Bray, came to see me. She examined me and told me that I was now in the hands of the "A Team." How right she was! This special team of two became a vital part of my life for the next twelve years. During my many hospitalizations for surgery and chemotherapy, and at the office, both Dr. Barton and Nancy were always available for me, as well as for the countless phone calls I have made over the years.

When a woman is faced with a diagnosis of cancer, having a supportive relationship with her physician and nurse, such as I had, can make a crucial difference in recovery. I was so fortunate to have all my care provided by my "A Team" and not in a clinic setting for chemotherapy, as many others are. I never felt alone during this "to hell and back" experience, as I knew I could always reach Dr. Barton or Nancy Bray.

I was beginning to have severe back pain and other discomforts, so during this time I was kept medicated with Dilaudid. I believe that sedation, plus the comfort I received from knowing that I had received two "negative ultrasounds," probably is what kept me from suspecting what truly was wrong with me.

Clinging to the false belief that my illness was not ovarian cancer, I asked Dr. Barton what he thought could be the problem. While I imagine he had no doubt in his mind, he never gave me cause to mistrust my beliefs. He said, "I won't know until I open you up." I accepted this and trusted him.

As I look back now on those five days, I still deeply ponder what kept me from sheer panic. It had to be more than just the effects of Dilaudid, Dr. Barton's reassurance, and my false beliefs about the ultrasounds. I recall that the nurses were noncommittal when I told them that "at least it's not ovarian cancer." I guess everyone knew except me. Intellectually, I should have known. I was usually a worrier and I always prided myself on my expert nursing knowledge, yet something that is beyond my understanding sustained me through this time of waiting and kept me from apprehension. Was I using denial as a defense mechanism already or was it, simply put, my faith in God that allowed me to relax and put myself in His hands?

During this period of waiting, I had several visits from a friend of many years, Dr. Robert (Pete) MacMillan. Pete is one of the few connections to my past professional nursing career at NEBH. He was a most respected physician who later became chief of staff and with whom I had kept in contact over the years. He reassured me that even if I had ovarian cancer, there were new treatments available. Of course, I told him that I couldn't have this horrible disease and reminded him of my "negative ultrasounds."

Surgery
Diagnosis: Ovarian Cancer

The day of my surgery finally arrived. It was February 10 when I made the trip to the operating room. Having been hospitalized for five days and medicated for pain, which kept me in a partial state of sedation, I didn't experience the preoperative jitters that most patients suffer. Even though I still clung to the belief that I didn't have ovarian cancer because my ultrasounds were "negative," I did have fears, fears of the unknown.

When I was prepared and on my way to the O.R., somehow I went peacefully with the blessings and loving care of the nurses on Lahey 5, the floor where I was a patient. In retrospect, I'm reasonably sure they all knew that I was about to enter the scary, painful domain of the cancer patient.

The four-hour surgical procedure for removal of the ovarian cancer that was found is known as debulking, or cytoreduction, in which all visible tumor is removed. In the beginning of the surgery, three liters of fluid were immediately removed from my abdomen. No wonder I felt bloated!

According to the operative report, there was tumor "studding the whole under-surface of the diaphragm." The omentum, which is a large fold of peritoneal layers that connect and support the internal organs of the abdomen, was involved and removed. Nodules were removed from the peritoneum, overlying both kidneys and ureters. The pelvis was "completely cemented in with tumor" and the terminal ileum, the end of the small bowel, had a massive tumor and was removed, along with about a foot of small intestine. The tumor encased the posterior surface of the bladder and this tumor was dissected. Tumor encased my whole recto-sigmoid and a resection of the sigmoid colon was done. Both ovaries were cancerous and, of course, removed, and a radical hysterectomy was also performed. My appendix was removed and many other things were removed or resected.

After everything was removed and examined by pathologists, the pathological staging was Stage III C ovarian cancer.

The surgery had been scheduled for early afternoon. Russ was urged to stay home and wait rather than be at the hospital, since he could not see me until the next day. Partway through the procedure, Nancy Bray left the operating room to call Russ and advise him of what was found and being done. Acknowledging that it was difficult to relay such news, especially by phone, she told him of my diagnosis with much compassion. Following the surgery, Dr. Barton phoned Russ with the details and gave him the encouragement he needed before he informed our children and my mother of the diagnosis and my condition.

I found out the diagnosis while still in the recovery room, but was sedated enough so that I didn't dwell on it for too long. The next day, back in my room, I bombarded the nurses with questions and was told that Dr. Barton would be in soon to talk with me. Knowing that I had ovarian cancer terrified me and I feared the worst. I had no idea how much tumor I had, how far it had spread, whether it had been "operable," or even if I would ever go home again.

I think I was more emotional than articulate in expressing my concerns, but Dr. Barton, in his gentle and compassionate way, answered my questions with honesty and reassurance. He explained to me that he had removed every bit of cancer that was visible and that he hoped the chemotherapy to follow would take care of what remained. He added that, "with the help of the Man Upstairs," I ought to do very well. I believed and trusted Dr. Barton and felt optimistic and grateful to be in his hands. I also became aware that we shared some sort of spiritual affirmation, and that was a comfort to me. When I had a few more days of recuperation, I would be ready to get on with the process of handling my diagnosis.

Russ came to visit every other day, and four days after my surgery was Valentine's Day. When he arrived he handed me a small, beautifully wrapped box. I was so dopey from pain medication that Russ helped me unwrap and open the box. Inside on a chain was a dainty silver pendant. Concealed within the design were the words, I LOVE YOU.

Of course, I was too bleary-eyed to really see it, but Russ described it to me. Since I still had tubes in my neck and my nose and was not ready to wear jewelry, Russ tucked it away safely in a drawer. When the day came that I was rid of some of my tubes and lines, Russ lovingly put the necklace on me and I shed my first tears—of joy and gratitude for his love.

Occasionally, Russ brought my mother to visit me. My illness smote her a mighty blow and she needed to see for herself how I was progressing. My father died when he was only sixty-eight, so my mother has been alone for many years. I have never fully gotten over losing my dad when I was still in my forties and needed him so much in my life. Our son, Jay, accompanied Russ a few times, but our daughters Nancy and Susan and their families were going through winter flu bugs, so we kept in touch through phone visits.

Each day I gained in strength and optimism, and the pain lessened as well. As more tubes and drains were removed, I was more mobile and walked around as much as I could.

I remained in the hospital for three weeks, then returned for chemotherapy every three or four weeks. Before chemotherapy, though, while I was recuperating and trying to handle my diagnosis, Dr. Barton suggested that a psychiatrist might help me to deal with my feelings a bit faster and easier. I told him I wasn't sure about that, but Dr. P., the psychiatrist, came in anyway. By then I had cleared my head fairly well. I made up my mind that I would fight and survive this disease. I told Dr. P. that I had a limited knowledge of imagery used in cancer treatment and planned to try it during my first chemotherapy, which was forthcoming.

I feel that each woman who is hospitalized for initial ovarian cancer treatment should have the option of some sort of counseling, be it pastoral or psychiatric, to help deal with her diagnosis. If she prefers to work things out in her own way and has support from loved ones, she may not need outside intervention.

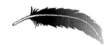

Working It Out

The Five Stages

Dr. Elisabeth Kübler-Ross, in *On Death and Dying,* explains the five stages of grief or of dealing with a terminal illness. These stages are coping mechanisms. When you have even a glimmer of hope that there can be some treatment available, by working through these different stages, coping becomes a lot easier.

The first stage is denial and isolation; the second, anger; the third, "bargaining"; the fourth, depression; and the fifth, acceptance. These stages go along with the loss of a loved one, a way of living with loss of a body part, or any extreme loss.

During the first stage of denial and isolation, I couldn't quite deny that I had ovarian cancer, but it was with utter disbelief and shock that I received this diagnosis. I had never been an ill person. I was very healthy, having jogged six or seven miles a day, and found it somewhat hard to believe that this could have happened to me, as I had been feeling so well.

Dr. Kübler-Ross explains that after the stage of denial passes, it is replaced by "feelings of anger, rage, envy, and resentment," with the next logical question being, "Why me?" This anger is difficult for others to deal with, as it is often displaced in many directions, including onto family and caregivers.

I remember this stage well. For some reason, I never shed a tear. I had numerous internal conflicts and thought of all the time that had been wasted by the failure to diagnose my cancer. I was angry to think that I might not be around to enjoy my family. Of course, I didn't know then if I was, in fact, dealing with a terminal illness, but from my frame of reference, I knew it was quite possible. I don't think that I was repressing my anger or overly displacing it; I was busy sorting out my feelings.

During this stage, I never asked "Why me?" Only much later in the course of my illness, when I had "no evidence of disease," did I say repeatedly but with different meaning, "Why me? Why did God choose to spare me?"

As far as envy—as part of the stage of anger—goes, I experienced it only much later when some of my residual physical limitations necessitated many changes in lifestyle. These changes, mostly related to my digestive dysfunctions, served as ever-present reminders of my cancer. There are events that are important to me, such as family gatherings and celebrations, special occasions with friends, concerts and athletic events involving our children and grandchildren, for which I made a great effort to attend. I did find myself envying others around me, who seemingly were healthy. For years Russ and I had regularly attended hockey games at the University of New Hampshire. I sometimes found myself scanning the crowd of thousands and wondering how many others were afraid of having an accident and not making it to the rest room. Was I the only one?

Impossible! Then reality stepped in and I looked around and realized how very blessed I was to be alive and healthy and under close medical scrutiny by the "best."

As to my rationalizations, everyone else could be a "walking time bomb" and not be aware of it. This was not meant to be an unkind thought, but it was probably true. I wouldn't wish again to be in anyone else's boots! Most sadly, I saw the devastating results of my conclusions, as over the last few years Russ and I have suffered the often sudden, unexpected losses of many dear friends, both young and old. I have never again felt envy.

I have no recollection of experiencing the stage of bargaining. Most of the bargains, according to Dr. Kübler-Ross, are made with God. I never tried to make a "deal" with Him, but I sure prayed a lot.

Somewhere between the stages of depression and acceptance I made a decision. Lying in that hospital bed, my mind went back to my home. "After I'm gone, who is going to be living there?" I wondered, "Who is going to take over as the 'lady of the house'? Who is going to be sharing my bedroom with my husband as a new wife? Certainly whoever it is isn't going to put up with that dark wallpaper that I have on the walls. What will happen to all of the foolish, dust-gathering, mundane things cluttering up the house—my thousands of antique marbles, baskets, wooden boxes, advertising whiskey tasters, and old medicine glasses?"

All of a sudden, I thought to myself, "The hell with this! I'm going to be there myself. I am not going to let this thing get me. I'm going to fight it and I'm going to make it and

I'm going to live!" And that was the turning point in my determination to survive.

During my brief visit with the psychiatrist, I had told him that I was beginning to feel comfortable with the way I was going to handle things and told him of my new, positive approach. He seemed to feel that it wasn't necessary for him to come back and was accepting of the way I was coping, so I didn't see him again.

Before I was due to be discharged, Dr. Barton suggested that I have my first chemotherapy treatment on a Tuesday and then I would go home the next day. He offered me this option, so that when I came home I would have experienced everything that there was to have experienced—and I did!

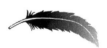

Toughing It Out

Chemotherapy

My first experience with imagery came about long before I ever thought it would become a regular part of my life. Several years before my illness with ovarian cancer, I had watched a television program dealing with children who were afflicted with terminal illnesses. With their very pliant minds and vivid imaginations, these children were able to use visualization or imagery in curing their tumors, using images such as Pac-Man, which was so popular at that time. They saw their cancer cells as some dreadful creatures and they were shooting them and killing them, and how very effective it was!

I was impressed by this, so when I had my first chemotherapy I decided that I would use a similar method, to see if I could enhance the effectiveness of the fluid that was going through my body during the initial stage of the chemotherapy. When it was done by an IV push, there wasn't too much I could do. But when the cisplatin hanging in the IV bottle first started dripping through my veins, I thought of it as a beautiful, sparkling, glistening miracle fluid going throughout every bit of my body, rather than the brutally toxic liquid that it is. I watched it on its way, killing off cancer cells, and I did this until the nausea and vomiting overtook me and I had to stop. But I do believe that I followed its healing path through every bit of my body first. And that was something I did throughout each session of chemotherapy.

I had all of my chemotherapy at the New England Baptist Hospital, directed by Dr. Barton, who is an oncological gynecologist. My protocol, known as CAP, consisted of cisplatin, Adriamycin, and Cytoxan. Since I needed to be hydrated with IV fluids for twenty-four hours, to which the chemotherapeutic drugs were added, and also during this time because I had severe nausea, vomiting, and diarrhea, I was hospitalized for a day for each one of these treatments.

My chemotherapy treatments were always on a Tuesday. How I dreaded them! Somehow, after each ordeal, I was able to put off worrying about the next treatment until two days before it was due. On Sunday morning, I began a twenty-four-hourly urine collection and on Monday I lugged my jug to the local hospital lab. There, I had a blood test to make sure that my white cell count was high enough and that my kidneys had suffered no damage, so I could have chemotherapy the next day.

Sitting in the admission office prior to one of the first few chemo treatments, I caught a glimpse of my admitting diagnosis, which was written on my medical record. When I saw the words "metastatic ovarian cancer," I felt sick inside. I knew my disease was advanced, but seeing the word "metastatic" devastated me. After I recovered sufficiently enough from this traumatic experience to think logically, I became more determined than ever to fight all the harder for my life.

All the way to Boston I was almost sick with fear, but I didn't say much. We only talked about how happy the ride home would be on Wednesday. After I was admitted and settled in my room, Russ would go home. I waited for my IV to be started and then the dreadful procedure would begin. The nurses and staff who cared for me during these deadly chemo sessions couldn't have been kinder or more attentive to my many needs. I was so sick that I vomited, had diarrhea, and wet the bed simultaneously. As soon as the nurses had me cleaned up and were headed for the door, I'd have a repeat performance. Usually, just before daybreak, I'd finally drift off to sleep for an hour.

When Dr. Barton and Nancy Bray came around seven a.m., I was eagerly waiting to be disconnected from my IV so I could go to the bathroom and brush my teeth. Amazingly, by then my nausea had subsided. I was ravenously hungry and able to enjoy a breakfast of orange juice, coffee, bacon, poached egg, and toast. After a comforting shower, I watched the clock waiting for Russ to come to take me home. What a joy to hear his footsteps approaching my room!

Most of the time, the drugs were still dripping through my veins during the evening hours and into the night. I found this very interesting when I began studying more about circadian rhythm and wondered if this timing, although it was coincidental, contributed in any way to my cure. I know that it was not planned this way, that it was just a matter of when therapy was started.

Circadian rhythm (from the Latin, meaning "around the day") alludes to the fact that the body's internal day of waking and sleeping is on a twenty-five- hour cycle, not twenty-four. It seems to indicate that timing the administration of chemotherapy, as well as other things in life, can be affected in the outcome. Understanding this cycle explains why it is easier to "spring ahead" in April than it is to set the clocks back an hour in the fall. We also find that we don't suffer jet lag as much flying west crossing other time zones as much as we do when flying east.

In the mid-eighties a physician at the University of Minnesota, Dr. William Hrushesky, conducted a study of sixty-two women with advanced ovarian cancer. Those who were treated at six in the morning and six in the evening had a remission rate three times that of those who were not given chemo at any specific time. (This study goes into a great deal more of the specifics as to how the survival was measured.) Another significant finding was that the patients who were given Adriamycin and cisplatin, as I was, on a particular schedule related to the circadian rhythm, had many fewer side effects and could tolerate larger doses than those in a random therapy group.

This may account for better remission rates. This enhancement of drug therapy could be because the drugs may have a more potent effect when hormone levels are higher and the tumor cells are dividing more rapidly.

Throughout my course of chemotherapy, I was carefully monitored for any damage to my heart and kidneys, since these potent drugs can be highly toxic to these organs. While many side effects were unpleasant, no permanent damage to my heart or kidneys occurred. Perhaps this success could be attributed, in part, to my circadian rhythm, even though it was unplanned.

Throughout the months that I was on chemotherapy, I had diarrhea much of the time, vomited often, and was quite content to lie around and not worry about getting things done. I was unable to eat most of the time, although breakfast usually was my best and most nourishing meal and one that I could usually keep down. About 5:30 a.m. I was wide awake and ravenous. I waited as long as I could, then prodded Russ. He prepared our breakfast until the actual egg-poaching moment—then I took over! Just as my appetite would return, it would be time to get whammed again with the next treatment.

One extreme side effect of the Adriamycin, was the development of mouth sores. This was very painful, and I got only slight relief from various topical medications; however, something worse was yet to come. I became unable to swallow—even liquids. Actually, liquids were harder to get down. My local physician, and good friend as well, Dr. Tom Clairmont, believed the problem to be a yeast infection. This was confirmed by a culture and treated effectively, although it did take time.

This infection had extended down my esophagus, and for three weeks I lived on my own ingenious concoctions, which could be swallowed more painlessly while maintaining my nutritional well-being. I drank apricot juice because it is bland and thick. I also mixed pureed baby meats with sour cream, which slid down fairly easily.

I remember thinking that, for once, I didn't need to worry about cutting down on fat and calories and secretly enjoyed the previously forbidden taste of the rich, creamy nectars. I even went so far as to tell my family that I'd never need to go on a diet again. How naive I was, yet how blessed I am, to have survived and now have the need to watch my weight!

I began to notice some tingling and numbness in my hands and feet, but not severe enough to concern me or to mention to Dr. Barton. By chance, I read an article in the *American Journal of Nursing*, November 1986, on the neurotoxicity of cisplatin, one of the drugs I had received. Most of the cases of peripheral neuropathy reported were more disabling than mine, and my symptoms diminished over time, although they remain to some degree. Reading this article eased my mind, explained what I had been experiencing, and reminded me once more how fortunate I was. Another article in the July 1987 *American Journal of Nursing*, discussed cisplatin neuropathy that worsened after exercise. For several years I experienced slight tingling and numbness after bowling or jogging.

During the seven months following my debulking surgery, I suffered several episodes of intestinal obstruction. These were due to the formation of adhesions. Each occurrence was painful, frightening, yet mercifully self-limiting. It would begin with intermittent abdominal pain, severe heartburn, and then the vomiting, which would eventually produce fecal material.

I knew that fecal vomiting meant that I was obstructed. This scared the bloody hell out of me! Such extreme vomiting would usually end with my fainting, and Russ would carry me to bed and revive me with an ammonia inhalant.

That would be the end of my obstruction until the next time it occurred. To be certain nothing more serious was causing these obstructions, I had an upper G.I. (gastrointestinal) series. The negative report was a great relief.

From then on, when I felt the first sign of an impending obstruction, I had the idea that perhaps I could prevent it by unkinking my intestine before it completely closed off. My method was rather offbeat: I was still fairly limber, so I leaned over the foot of the bed, put my hands on the floor, and had Russ lift both of my legs so that I ended up standing on my head. I'm not sure how effective this maneuver was but on one occasion I do think the attack was less severe, although it was probably "all in my head." When I mentioned this to Dr. Barton and to Dr. Clairmont, they smiled and probably thought I was not serious. During my second-look surgery, the adhesions were lysed (loosened) and I had no more episodes of intestinal obstruction.

Despite so many side effects from the toxic drugs, I somehow kept from becoming too discouraged, although some days were brutal. Nancy Bray told me she believed that "the harder it all hits you, the better the job it is doing killing cancer cells." I agree!

Support Systems

Throughout these months, I know that support from my family and friends and prayers from prayer groups in my home area, contributed toward my healing. I have many friends from the University of New Hampshire hockey group and I was told that the UNH hockey team beat the britches off one of our greatest rivals one night while I was in the hospital because the coach, Charlie Holt, said, "You win this one for Barbara!" Later, the team presented me with a hockey stick autographed with all the players' names. That was inspirational, knowing that the UNH hockey team was all out there skating for me.

Our very special friends, Ruth and Rip Therrian, sent frequent cards and notes of encouragement and always filled me in on the inside news of our UNH hockey team. Because of our mutual love of the animals in our lives, they always had an adventure to relate about their pets or sent clippings they knew would make me chuckle. Ruth is one who doesn't think I'm a nut because I've given CPR to a few chipmunks who had the misfortune to end up in our pool.

We have a good friend, a retired physician, Dr. Tom Chretien, who said to me once, "Barbara, don't ever let yourself think for one minute that you won't make it." I have remembered those words and believed very strongly in what he said. In encouraging so many other cancer patients I have met on this journey and tried to help, I always pass along that quote from Doc—it was so meaningful to me.

During this time I was truly blessed with the loving-kindness of many caring friends. I also received notes and cards from people I hadn't heard from in years.

A special treat during this time, when I was not able to handle dining out, was dinner at the home of Bobby Jean and Barton Seekins. Bobby and I had been friends and nursing colleagues for many years and fought our way through college together after our children were all in school. Their home was one of the few refuges, other than the homes of our family, where I could feel comfortable and not worry about embarrassing myself with an unexpected G.I. catastrophe.

I always felt at ease, too, with lifelong friends Paul and Carolyn Harvey, who were always there for me with loving support, flowers, food, and prayers. So many friends provided me with both spiritual and edible sustenance. They brought me casseroles and put me on their church prayer lists. Oh, how very blessed I was and am!

One friend of ours who had a life-threatening experience nearly coinciding with mine, chose to keep her illness from others, and I often wonder how anyone can cope and survive without the loving support of friends and close neighbors. While this is a personal choice, I would encourage those who are diagnosed with cancer to share the experience and allow others to participate in their recovery, at least with our prayers for healing.

One of the greatest loves in my life was Kim, our Siamese cat. He played a most important role on my healing journey. About the same time as my "fibroid" was discovered, Kim, at the age of seven, developed a serious eye problem. We took him to Dr. Alan Bachrach, a veterinary ophthalmologist who treated him surgically but, due to a complexity of problems, Kim gradually lost his sight. He developed glaucoma, and we administered his eye drops twice daily and took him for regular checkups.

Kim eventually lost all vision, but he managed amazingly well. As Dr. Bachrach told us, "Kim didn't wake up one day and think, 'Wow! I'm blind.' " Besides, Kim didn't need to read or drive. "He should do well," the doctor said. He did.

I missed Kim tremendously while I was hospitalized and couldn't wait to get home to hug him and figure out how he'd treat me. He'd sometimes be standoffish because I had left him; at other times he would greet me lovingly, wrapping his tail around my legs, and turn up his purr motor to HIGH. However he welcomed me, it didn't take him long to find me either on the couch or in bed. After the initial pounce, he would plunk his warm, furry little self on my tummy and be my comforting heating pad. After my soreness decreased, his presence was even more welcome.

One positive aspect of our frequent trips to Dr. Bachrach, whose office is in Lincoln, Massachusetts, was that these rides made a traveler out of a cat who had previously howled his throaty Siamese head off as soon as we left our driveway. Kim's new attitude allowed us to take him with us on most of the trips to our Berkshire house, where this "seacoast kitty" became a "Berkshire kitty" until we returned home. Even without his sight, Kim adapted well to these temporary changes in his residence and always found where his special places were, particularly our bed.

He will always have a special place in our hearts, while, since 1992, he rests under a white quartz stone from the Berkshires in our seacoast garden.

Body Image
The Crowning Glory

Before I was discharged from the hospital after my debulking surgery and first chemotherapy treatment, Dr. Barton and Nancy Bray visited me with instructions and explanations of what I could expect. Nancy told me that chemotherapy would cause me to lose my hair. She suggested that I take time to look for a good wig early in the loss process so it would be available when I needed it. I had guessed this would happen, but had never brought it up. Wishful thinking on my part that perhaps my locks would be spared!

Body image is very important, especially at a time when you have so many things to fight for and worry about. While it might not seem to be a major concern, losing your hair can be a very traumatic experience.

One thing that was very helpful to me was not having to look at the handfuls of it falling out. Once it was all gone it was easier to deal with than was the process of losing it. To see clumps daily in the bottom of the shower was not pleasant. Russ, bless his heart, did much to ease these anxieties. Each morning as I got up he would quickly vacuum the hair that had accumulated on my pillow so I wouldn't have to look at this symbol of my disease.

I have a story about my wigs. I made a mistake by going to a shop that had been recommended to me to buy a wig. It was a pretty tired-looking shop and I bought a pretty tired-looking wig before all of my hair was gone. I put the wig aside until I knew I would have to go somewhere and look respectable, instead of just wrapping a bandanna around my head, which was getting pinker and balder every day.

The first time I left the house for a social event was in the spring. This was the UNH hockey banquet and I went with a great deal of trepidation. I got dressed, relaxing a bit knowing that the restaurant wasn't too far away. As the final detail, I put the wig on—and recoiled in sheer horror at what I saw in the mirror. I looked like "Mama," Vicki Lawrence's role in the Carol Burnett Show, and it was perfectly dreadful. I ripped it off and said, "No way am I going anywhere in this thing!"—but I did.

I went to the hockey banquet and was touched by the hundreds of people there who joined in a special prayer led by my dear friend, the late Ruth Rowell, to welcome me back and wish me Godspeed in my recovery. From then on, I thought, "I can't do much about this wig—I'll stay home." That was not good—a very negative attitude on my part.

I looked through the Yellow Pages and found, much to my great joy, a beauty shop that advertised wigs in a town a short distance away. I plopped my foolish-looking wig over my head and rode to the shop. I walked in and a young gentleman greeted me, saying, "Can I help you?" I asked him if they sold wigs and he said, "No, we no longer carry wigs, but I think I know what your problem is and could help you if you wish. Would you like me to trim and shape that wig for you?" Of course I was delighted, and made my way to his chair.

I suppose he took pity on me because he then said, "How would you like a free makeup?" So I thought, "Why not let him pamper me?" I didn't watch him in the mirror. I thought I'd wait until he finished and be surprised. He worked and applied his talents for some time. He gave me what I think might be called an eyebrow arch. He worked and worked and worked. When I finally looked in the mirror, I was speechless. My lips had never been so red, my eyebrows so fine and defined. I was made up and looked like what we used to call a "painted whore"—guess this dates me. I thanked him profusely and told him what a lovely job he had done and that I felt sure my husband would be just thrilled to take me out to dinner that night.

I got in the car and headed home cautiously, thinking that if I was stopped, the police might think I had been out soliciting. I stopped by to see Bobby Jean and Bart and said, "Look at me now, because you'll never see me like this again." When I got home, my husband took one look at me and we really had a good laugh.

I'm not sure what the outcome would have been had I not had this cosmetological makeover, as far as my loss of brows and lashes. I may have kept my eyebrows; but when I tried to remove the "goop" from my eyelashes, my eyelashes came off with it.

After wondering for years where my son (and one of his sons as well) got his double-crowned head of hair, I discovered the source; I found that I, too, am double-crowned.

As my bald head received its signal that chemotherapy was concluded and it was okay to begin sprouting, it was easy to get to the "root" of my hair and discover the crowns and cowlicks I had always wondered about. These tiny spears of hair developed slowly and wondrously into tight curls.

In the meantime, I did find a really nice wig, which made a great difference in my appearance and my morale. I know that my attempt to keep looking well pleased Dr. Barton because he told me about one of his patients who would not bother to cover her bald head and took no interest in her appearance. He said that her indifference offended him. I was pleased that I was able to keep up my appearance to the best of my ability, as my endurance would allow—at least in public. A positive self-image can do wonders for keeping up morale.

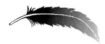

CA 125

Prior to my surgery, I had a blood test called a CA 125. The CA 125 measures the presence of ovarian tumor antigen, which is present in about 80 percent of patients who have ovarian cancer. The CA 125 measures the tumor markers. This test can produce false positive or false negative results due to a variety of factors, so it is not a reliable screening test, but it is extremely vital in monitoring the treatment of patients who have ovarian cancer.

A normal CA 125 is from 0 to 35. My initial count prior to surgery was 266. After my first chemotherapy treatment it dropped to 29. This significant plummet is considered to be a good predictor of prognosis. My next CA 125, following my second chemotherapy treatment, was "less than 5," where it has remained. (At times it has been reported as "too small to be measured.") The CA 125 has been a part of each checkup I have with Dr. Barton every three months. After completing nine years with NED (no evidence of disease) written on my record at each visit, I graduated to a CA 125 every six months.

This test is an expensive laboratory procedure and I went through an incredible and prolonged battle with my insurance company for reimbursement of the charges. To those women who may have been refused payment on the premise that the CA 125 is experimental, I can say unequivocally that this is not true. I conducted a medical library computer search on CA 125, the results of which enabled me to challenge our insurance carrier. And I won!

As I mentioned, the CA 125 is not a valid or reliable screening process. While it was being investigated as a possible tool for screening, insurance companies may have thought that every woman, living in fear of developing ovarian cancer, would inundate the laboratories to be tested at their expense. This is only one of my theories as to why I had such a difficult time persuading my insurance company to reimburse me. For those of us ovarian cancer patients, any elevation in the CA 125 would sound the alert that something was brewing and give us a head start to search for the cause. Our lives could depend on it!

The Summer of '86

That summer of 1986 had been a tough struggle for me, and I was counting the days until my course of chemotherapy would be finished. Just the thought of not having to endure what felt like torture kept me going. There were many events, common to a summer on the seacoast with family and friends, that I would have enjoyed participating in more fully if I'd had the strength and not been experiencing nausea and diarrhea most of the time. I did submit to permitting myself indulgence in being lazy without worrying or feeling guilt. I accepted the fact that my body was allowing the chemotherapy to do its job of healing me and realized that it was a full-time job.

While I was recuperating, our son, Jay, moved in with us from June into September while his new house was being built in Maine. Having him back here was a happy time, and I did have a chance to help him with his house and a bit of decorating.

As Jay was a bachelor at the time, and had no desire to invest in expensive furniture, I was able to help furnish his new home by refinishing a few nice old pieces. He had a dining table and had rescued four old chairs that someone had considered to be "dumpworthy." Seeing their potential, as the wood and the workmanship were good, I had them set up in our garage and mustered up enough energy to spend an hour or so each day refinishing these chairs for him. I was delighted with the results and the soft satin finish I had created. I bought an upholstery fabric to blend with his decor and Jay was most pleased. Being able to accomplish something worthwhile was a good feeling for me.

In 1990, Jay married Joanne, and the chairs are still being used in the dining room of their new home. I told them, "Don't you ever dare get rid of these chairs—they are one of my few good memories of the summer of 1986."

Both our daughters, Nancy and Susan, and their families lived in the area and were most supportive. I enjoyed the loving visits and special times spent with our two granddaughters. Nancy's Lindsay was three and Susan's Sarah was seven at the time. My mother was also a great help, living only a mile away. She was eighty years old and still driving, so she would do errands, shop for groceries, cook something special to tempt my appetite, or just sit with me when I felt so sick.

This same summer, another event became a part of our daily lives. The focus of this was a large, ungainly creature known as the *USS Albacore* (AGSS 569). This submarine became the "other woman" in my life because the job of putting her on display as a museum for the public had been a commitment made by my husband, prior to my illness, during the year before he retired.

This submarine had been in mothballs since its decommissioning in 1972 and the project developed into much more than we bargained for. My knowledge of the boat grew as I was kept entertained, lying on the couch, listening to the numerous phone calls Russ made to various parts of the country to locate and arrange for delivery of parts.

I became engrossed in the retrieval of the two propellers that had been left behind in Philadelphia when *Albacore* was towed to Portsmouth. When they actually arrived on a huge flatbed trailer one warm humid evening, Russ took me to an isolated area behind a storage warehouse where we could see them and touch them. They were really here after an exasperating exercise in logistics.

Being married to a submarine design engineer since 1953, I was quite familiar with these unique vessels; however, I never expected I'd swab the decks of one of them—but I did. *Albacore* was to have its grand opening that Labor Day weekend. It was unusually warm and humid, a bad wig day, so I tied on my bandanna and off we went to spiff up the big whale for its presentation to the community. It's amazing what we can accomplish when we're motivated. I guess it was patriotism that stirred me to move.

I had my final chemotherapy early in August, so I celebrated the culmination of two important events.

Labor Day was behind us and the tourists left. The beaches were now ours, and walking along the shore became more enjoyable and healing to me. Russ and I were walking the beach one early fall day and I felt quite lighthearted, digging my toes into the wet sand and then watching the tide come in and obliterate my footprints. In a whimsical mood, I picked up a seagull feather and stuck it in my wig, saying, "Here I am—the old Nokomis herself."

(I had recently found an old book in our Berkshire house in Cummington, *The Complete Poems of Henry Wadsworth Longfellow,* and reread "The Story of Hiawatha" with much enjoyment and nostalgia.)

Then, a bit more solemn, I said to Russ, "Now that my chemo is finished, if I have a 'clean' second-look surgery in September and work hard on my own to truly lick this rotten disease, it will really be a feather in my cap."

Russ looked at me and said, "You'll do it! For now, though, you'll have to settle for a feather in your wig."

Second Look

The end of September, I returned to the New England Baptist Hospital for a "second-look" laparotomy, and at this time the adhesions responsible for the intestinal obstructions were lysed. Adhesions are an abnormal sticking together of organs, usually intestines, occurring occasionally after abdominal surgery. Lysing involves releasing these abnormalities. I was roused from my post-anesthesia nap by the nurses excitedly telling me that I was "clean." That there was no tumor left was a sign that the surgery and the chemotherapy had been successful. The pathology report on the fluid in my abdomen read, "No tumor cells found."

This was a pleasant hospital stay, even shorter than I expected. My surgery took place on a Wednesday afternoon, and when I heard that Russ and my daughter Nancy were coming to visit Saturday morning, I decided that I'd like to return home with them. I could usually predict the exact time that Dr. Barton and Nancy Bray would visit me during their morning rounds, so I dragged myself out of bed, put on lipstick and my bandanna, and waited until I heard the familiar footsteps coming down the hall. Then, in a nightie and robe instead of the old johnny, I forced myself to stand up straight and greeted Dr. Barton halfway down the hall by doing a little "soft shoe" dance.

After my performance, followed by an examination, Dr. Barton said, "I think you want to go home." I assured him that I did, and asked when I could leave. He said, "How about today?" I was packed and on the phone within seconds, telling Russ to pick up Nancy quickly, never mind visiting me, but just be ready to bring me home.

Although it was barely lunchtime, I insisted that we stop for a meal on the way home. Always ready and eager to celebrate any of my triumphs, I had a cocktail and, being in an Italian restaurant, indulged in all I could of its culinary specialties. Not bad for my third post-op day! I was ready to proceed with living the rest of my life to its fullest.

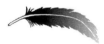

The Healing Journey

The Mind-Body
Connection and Imagery

I began my healing, both physical and emotional, at the moment when I was declared free of all disease. I decided that my life didn't depend totally on fate, or completely with the medical profession. I realized that I needed to participate and do my part as well. It was at this time that I decided how I would wage my war against this disease and never allow complacency to enter. I began my personal and continuing healing methods.

This healing journey began by reading many books on the mind-body connection and alternative healing. I would use these practices only as a supplement to the outstanding medical care I was receiving from Dr. Barton. The first book I read was Dr. Bernie Siegel's *Love, Medicine and Miracles*. I also borrowed his videotape from our local hospital and gained more insight into being what Dr. Siegel describes as an "exceptional patient."

Dr. Joan Borysenko, former cellular biologist and cofounder/former director of the Mind/Body Clinic in Boston, inspired me to delve more into the wonders of how powerfully the mind affects the body through her book *Minding the Body, Mending the Mind*. Several years later, I attended one of her lectures and participated in a professional healthcare workshop that she conducted.

Dr. Herbert Benson's *The Relaxation Response* and also *Beyond the Relaxation Response* started my daily ritual of meditating, even before my illness, and has remained with me through these many years.

During the months of chemotherapy, I had not really developed any particular imagery, except what I was able to use while having the actual treatment. I knew that since I was free of disease, I needed to develop a belief system tied in with a program of imagery that I would design to keep my immune system so strong that no cancer cells could ever enter my body. This imagery has become an integral part of my life.

In developing my belief system and imagery, I began with a review of the immune system so that I could design my imagery in a quasi-scientific manner. Actually, much of my visualization fell into place by appearing from my subconscious mind in an unexpected way, much better than I could have contrived. Psychoneuroimmunology, or PNI, is a term given by psychologist Robert Ader. A discipline arising during the 1970s, PNI explains how the brain and the mind can cause us to be ill or healthy. Ader inserted "neuro" in the middle of the term "psychoimmunology." This science that links the mind and the immune system was discovered by immunologist, Dr. Alfred Amkraut and psychiatrist, George Solomon.

The effect of the mind on the immune system has been the subject of much research centering on biochemicals called neuropeptides. These are hormonal messengers secreted by the brain, the immune system, and nerve systems in various other organs.

Our endocrine glands secrete hormones that control every tissue and organ in the body. This hormone mixture is controlled by the pituitary, also known as the master gland. It is located just below the brain in the head, but the output of hormones from this master gland is controlled by secretions and nerve impulses from the hypothalamus.

The hypothalamus is a very small part of the brain. It regulates most of the body functions over which we have no conscious control such as temperature, heart rate, blood pressure, and breathing. The emotional center of the brain is called the limbus or the limbic area, and what we feel emotionally controls the action of the hypothalamus.

Numerous nerves connect the hypothalamus to all parts of the immune system—the thymus, the spleen (where dwell our white blood cells) the lymph glands, the whole lymph system. Understanding this, we know that there is direct control of our immune system by our brain.

Much has been written over the past ten or fifteen years about the mind/body connection. I think it's important to have this understanding of the immune system in order to believe in the healing power of imagery.

Imagery was first used to treat cancer by oncologist O. Karl Simonton and Stephanie Matthews-Simonton, who was then his wife. They were the first Western practitioners to use imagery in the healing or treatment of cancer. In their book *Getting Well Again*, written with James Creighton, the Simontons say that the common thread running through these disciplines is that people created mental images of desired events.

According to Belleruth Naparstek, a psychotherapist and author of *Staying Well with Guided Imagery*, images in the mind can be almost as real as the actual event.

We all use imagery, whether or not we are aware of it. When we read a book, we create images in our minds of the scenes and characters about whom we are reading; yet each of us has a distinct, unique picture.

For example, a story may begin in a small white farmhouse at the end of a dirt road. Next to the old house are the remains of a partially collapsed barn. While this scene seems quite clear and ordinary, no two people could picture it in their minds exactly the same way. Many times it is a disappointment to see a movie after enjoying the book from which the movie was adapted because nothing appears the way we had visualized it.

Another example of imagery occurs involuntarily when the thought of a particular food enters our minds, such as when we think of crunching into a red, juicy apple or sucking on a sour lemon. How easy it is to feel your hands grow red and tingle with cold as you remember scooping up fresh heavy snow without gloves and molding it into a snowball.

Children are endowed with incredible imaginations. Their minds are virtual receptacles of the most intriguing imagery. I remember watching, unobserved, with amazement as my children (and now my grandchildren) became engrossed in "pretend" games.

Many children grow up with an "imaginary" playmate. Our daughter Susan had such a friend. Her name was Dorothy Reynolds and she often accompanied our family on day trips. We even knew where she lived and what her home was like, although we never did actually see it. Then, too, children have no problem seeing "boogie men" after the lights are out at night and can describe the funny little elves that wake them early in the morning.

Visiting with cancer patients who were friends or acquaintances, or with women who were recently diagnosed and sought me out, I tried to help them with the new experience of imagery. To illustrate what imagery is all about, I shared an audiotape that I had made. To some, I could tell that my imagery sounded pretty "far out." One friend who had non-Hodgkin's lymphoma had been struggling in her attempt to visualize polar bears gobbling up the cancer cells within her. After listening to my tape, she said, "I think that I'm just too inhibited to let myself really get into this imagery thing."

It is so important to realize that imagery is our very own personal experience. It rises from our subconscious, yet we can mold it and direct it to fulfill our needs. We cannot compare it to that of anyone else, nor can we allow others to "design" it for us—they can only guide us in finding our own images.

Guardian Angels and Inner Guides

The Simontons wrote that an Inner Guide allows us to open the door to the unconscious, which holds priceless healing powers. Through the Inner Guide, a person is able to carry on conversations, receiving answers to questions that "seem to be beyond the individual's conscious capabilities." The Inner Guide frequently appears in the form of an authoritative figure or a religious being.

Dr. Gerald Epstein, in his book *Healing Visualizations or Creating Health Through Imagery,* describes "inner guides" who, in the Western spiritual tradition, appear to be angels. They are referred to throughout the Bible (both the Old and the New Testaments) and the Koran and are mentioned in Christianity, Islam, and Judaism. These three spiritual traditions mention that we are all born with a guardian angel and can summon this guardian angel whenever we want its presence. This angel can appear in many ways. It could be in human form, in animal form, or as a creature from another world—however we want to perceive this inner guide or guardian angel.

This supposition is most interesting to me since I had not been aware of this revelation when I created my imagery. The exuberant little creature who bounded into my imagery and into my life called himself Thaddeus. Thaddeus, who has been the leader of my troupe, whom I refer to as my TLC guys, is my Inner Guide. TLC in the nursing vernacular stands for "tender loving care," and also relates to T-lymphocyte cells, most important in the immune system. I never considered why the name Thaddeus jumped out to me from my subconscious, but later the reason became clear.

Several times in my life I have suffered extreme anguish of both body and spirit. Joan Borysenko describes what she calls a "dark night of the soul" in her book *Fire in the Soul*. Billy Graham, in *Angels*, recalled a time when he felt alone and deserted with these trials and burdens, a "dark night for my soul." During these dark nights of my soul when all else failed, I called upon St. Jude to intercede. This saint of the hopeless is actually St. Jude Thaddeus, friend of Jesus. I believe this is why my spiritual or inner guide appeared to me bearing the name of Thaddeus.

Because Thaddeus has been a vital part of my life these last twelve years, I would like to elaborate on the life of this somewhat obscure biblical character whose namesake has chosen to spend his life with me. In material sent to me from the St. Jude shrine, I read that during the fourteenth century, Jesus came to St. Bridget in a vision and told her to pray to St. Jude, telling her that "in accordance with his surname 'Thaddeus' (meaning amiable and loving) he will show himself most willing to help."

Not being very knowledgeable about saints, I found the story in an old booklet from my children's Sunday school days more comforting. This booklet, called *The Twelve Apostles* by Loice Gouker, explains that this particular disciple had many names, among them Jude, Judas (not to be confused with the twelfth disciple, Judas Iscariot, who betrayed Jesus), Labbaeus, and Thaddeus.

According to this story, Abgarus, the King of Edessa, became ill. Hearing of the miraculous healing powers of Jesus, Abgarus sent for Him to come and heal him. Supposedly, Jesus answered, telling Abgarus, "It is necessary that those things for which I was sent should be completed, after which I shall be received up to Him who sent me. When, therefore, I shall be received into heaven, I shall send one of my disciples who shall heal you." So Jude is said to have been sent "in due time." Jude was supposed to have been a great traveler overseas and his symbol in art is a sailboat, representing his travels to Edessa, Syria, Arabia, and Mesopotamia in his healing work for Christ.

Thaddeus, my Inner Guide or Spiritual Guide is not my guardian angel. I do have a real true guardian angel who has rescued me from many near-disastrous situations. I know in my heart that it was my guardian angel assigned by God that sent Dr. Barton to me.

Billy Graham said that the existence of angels is mentioned in the Bible more than three hundred times. He quotes Martin Luther, who said, "An angel is a spiritual creature created by God without a body for the service of Christendom and the church." Dr. Graham explains that we are not always aware of the angels' presence, but they could be our neighbors or our companions without our knowledge. Many of us believe that we have been helped through the ministrations of angels, while others are not aware of the assistance given to them by angels performing the duties assigned to them by God.

During several close calls, when some tragedy has been miraculously averted, I always thank God, and I really believe I am thanking Him for sending my guardian angel in the nick of time to protect me or my loved ones. Over these past twelve years, my guardian angel has manifested its presence more often, perhaps because my physical condition has been more precarious, although I have felt this divine presence many times during my life.

On one occasion many years ago, when I was a charge nurse on a busy floor before the days of recovery rooms, I had an experience I'll always remember. I was sitting at my desk engrossed in my duties when, for some unknown reason, I felt something draw me to the room of a patient who had undergone thyroid surgery a few hours earlier. I ran to her bedside and found her hemorrhaging and in respiratory distress, only minutes after she had been checked by the nurse caring for her. No doubt my intervention saved her life, but I believe either her guardian angel or mine took me to her bedside.

In fighting to survive ovarian cancer, remember that you are never alone; you have a guardian angel to guide you through the dark hours.

"God has delegated himself to a million deputies."
—Ralph Waldo Emerson

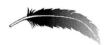

Thaddeus, the Immune System, and My Imagery

Thaddeus, my Inner Guide, is a T-cell. The immature T-stem cells are derived from bone marrow. During fetal development, they move to the thymus, where they undergo a very complicated series of maturation events until they become mature T-lymphocytes. The thymus is a small gland located behind the sternum, or breastbone. These T-cells leave the thymus and are found in parts of the blood, traveling through their very own lymphatic system to watch over the body. They are concentrated in lymph nodes and in the spleen. This is the important immune system on which I base my imagery.

I began using imagery to supplement conventional therapy following my initial surgery, chemotherapy, and second-look surgery. It was, and still is, aimed at strengthening my immune system to prevent a recurrence of cancer. I describe my type of visualization as being passionate imagery, because I envision my killer T-cells as triathletes. I am a jogger myself and, rather than do my daily imagery in a conventional state of relaxation, I practice it in a more stimulating situation while I run, walk, or ride a bicycle.

Occasionally, I do sit in a meditative mood and go through my imagery, particularly if I am riding in the car. I don't adhere strictly to scientific facts because I believe that imagery should be more symbolic, and you should strive to be comfortable knowing that your belief system is suited to meet your individual needs.

While my imagery is, in many ways, considered to be "receptive imagery" because, according to Barbara Dossey, the images "seem to just 'bubble up' ", it is also "active imagery." It is active in that after Thaddeus manifested himself to me, we developed a close relationship involving dialogue, emotional support and guidance in nearly all aspects of daily life.

To the uninitiated, my personal experience with imagery may seem off the wall, but to those of you who are living through a cancer episode, this baring of my soul may help in developing your own imagery. While mine is aimed at preventing recurrence, those currently battling the disease should direct their efforts to killing off the cancer cells. Work at picturing them as some sort of dreadful creatures and fantasize them as being eliminated in some sort of atrocious manner. Kill them off in any dramatic way that your imagination can conjure up that is acceptable to your belief system.

There are many theories as to why cancer develops. A very interesting theory, according to Dr. Bernie Siegel, and one widely accepted is called "The Surveillance Theory of Cancer." This states that cancer cells are developing in our bodies all the time and are destroyed by the white blood cells normally before they become tumors. Cancer appears when the immune system becomes suppressed and can't deal with whatever is upsetting it, so the emotional part of the brain, which controls the immune system, fosters the cancer.

Since I live under stress, as most people do, my immune system is being kept strong with my imagery. Also, because this time set aside to practice imagery is a happy experience, my hypothalamus is positively affecting my immune system. Thaddeus pushes a button within my inner self, known only to him and to me, and that part of my brain strengthens and gives an added push to all parts of my immune system.

We now know how the immune system works against cancer. The immune system is very complicated, so I will simplify it as best as I can. The human body has two types of immunity. One is known as humoral immunity, which depends on antibodies present in the body fluids that fight off infection. The other immune system, called cell-mediated immunity, fights off viruses and tumors. It is this type of defense system that I will concentrate on because it composes the T-lymphocytes, or the T-cells, which play a great role in killing cancer cells.

Thaddeus and his glorious horde of TLC guys are tiny pixielike creatures with pinkish white heads, shaped like the letter T. Their bodies are pink and their faces are indistinct except for two impish eyes and a smile.

My imagery begins with a daily greeting among me, Thaddeus and the rest of the group, with reassurance that both I and my immune system are in great shape, and that I have been totally scanned and monitored constantly, day and night, by this instrument inside me that is so far beyond state-of-the-art that medical science could not believe it was possible.

I then ask for a computer readout showing the present

state of my immune system. At that very moment Thaddeus steps from the multitude of the "guys," pushes a button, and across the screen flashes a big smile followed by "No cancer cells present, clean as a whistle," at which point the whole gang whistles. (Do I sound like a nut case yet?) Then it says, "Cured of all malignancy forever and immune to all malignancy forever." We comment on our great fortune and success.

Next Thaddeus zaps my thymus to ensure that we always have just the right kind of cells "on call." By pulling a lever, he sends a surge of a powerful biochemical throughout my entire body, my circulatory system, immune system, the lymphatic system, spleen, thymus, and bone marrow. This marvelous chemical is pulsating and swishing throughout me. I can feel this vital liquid on its journey throughout every bit of my body, empowering me to believe that I am impervious to a recurrence of disease. Thaddeus and I then agree that I have the strongest immune system in all of creation. It is then that Thaddeus explains how he and his TLC guys keep me so strong.

First, they meditate. Then they do these marvelous strengthening exercises and proceed to what we call the Platinum Man Triathlon. When they participate in their daily Platinum Man Triathlon, their apparel changes. For the footrace they wear running shoes, shorts, and tank tops with a big "T" on the front and the back. When they jump into the vast expanse of water to swim, they are seen briefly in trunks. Then they immerse too quickly to be observed any further. For the bike ride, helmets shaped like a "T" cover their strange little heads, biking pants and tops are added, and away they go. They run four hundred miles, swim three hundred miles, and bike five hundred miles. Then, to my utter amazement, they reverse the event and go back the same way they came.

In our dialogue, I say to them, "This is incredibly incredible," and Thaddeus says, "Yes, but this symbolizes the extraordinary strength of your immune system, Barbara."

This is followed by what I call my "message for the day," in which I receive a lecture from Thaddeus. Sometimes this includes a pat on the back or a kick in the rear, but always one message stays the same. It is how to live my life, what's important and what's not—how to deal with stresses and how to count my blessings.

Most of my early experiences with Thaddeus and his group have remained essentially the same. On several occasions, when I was hospitalized for surgery and unable to visualize as usual, I would call on Thaddeus long enough to tell him that it was up to him to keep tabs on me and give my immune system its daily zapping until I could take charge again. My imagery always ends with a time of prayerful thanksgiving to God for my loving family, friends, and Dr. Barton.

This daily spiritual journey is vital to my existence— the true self-nurturance. It is a time to put worries and foolish trivialities to rest and to retrieve the positive attitude that has helped me to survive.

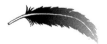

The Blessings of
a Positive Attitude

When we are at the pinnacle of our productive and healthy years and tragedy strikes, when we are experiencing pain, as well as physical, emotional, and social losses, it is beyond our grasp to believe that anything good can arise from these adversities.

But many blessings have come my way as the result of my misfortune. If I had not had ovarian cancer, numerous opportunities to enrich my life would have been missed. There are relationships that never would have been developed, and special soul-baring moments from others afflicted with this dreadful disease would not have been shared with me. I have had renewed friendships with acquaintances and associates from past years, and have enjoyed closer ties with my family.

To think that I never would have been privileged to know Dr. Barton or gain a special friend in Nancy Bray is a devastating thought. I also discovered many things about Russ: not only his loving support and devotion, but also his ability to help me out of some situations that could easily have sent a lesser man running in the opposite direction.

Ralph Waldo Emerson wrote, "For everything you have missed, you have gained something else; and for everything you gain, you lose something."

By holding the belief that no cancer cells can ever enter my body again, I have developed a philosophy that is not based on fear or "what-ifs," or, as some cancer patients believe, that there is "not much I can do about it. If it comes back, it comes back."

As a result of my belief system, I have not allowed myself to worry, at least consciously, about recurrence. I know that for a few days prior to my checkups with Dr. Barton every three months, I experience various minor psychosomatic ailments; at least, my husband tells me I'm not quite myself. I guess I gripe more than usual and feel like I'm falling apart physically and emotionally. Yet consciously I am never afraid of Dr. Barton giving me bad news. Dr. Barton suggested once that it must be a tense time for me, but in all honesty, except for that brief moment when my humanness surpasses my moxie during my exam, I know that I am well. If I allowed myself to think otherwise, my whole belief system, symbolized by my imagery, would be a useless exercise.

While I don't want to give the impression of being a Pollyanna, it is this attitude of positive thinking, trust, and hope that I believe has contributed to my survival of ovarian cancer without recurrence. This is what has helped me to endure the many painful physical and emotional experiences of my life these last twelve years. Dr. Larry Dossey, in his book *Meaning and Medicine,* says, "The dominant message" incessantly preached from the editorial pages of medical journals or the podiums of medical schools is that "the inherent biology of the disease is overwhelmingly important in that feelings, emotions, and attitudes are simply along for the ride."

I first practiced meditation several years before my experience with cancer. I learned the technique from reading Dr. Herbert Benson's book *The Relaxation Response*. As a novice, I had much to learn. Particularly, I needed to know how to find quiet, private, uninterrupted time during a busy day. I solved this problem quite simply by closing the door, taking the phone off the hook, and putting the cat outside. I discovered I could attain a meditative state quite well. My mind and body responded remarkably in that I was able to return to my daily activities with a heightened sense of well-being.

When Dr. Benson's *Beyond the Relaxation Response* was published, I advanced to this method using what he calls the "faith factor." The Relaxation Response refers to the innate ability of the body to enter a special state that offsets the harmful effects of stress and involves: "(1) finding a quiet environment; (2) consciously relaxing the body's muscles; (3) focusing for ten to twenty minutes on a mental device such as the word one or a brief prayer; and (4) assuming a passive attitude toward intrusive thoughts."

After several years, Dr. Benson came to believe that there was more required to achieve optimal benefit from the Relaxation Response. This new understanding resulted in his belief that combining the Relaxation Response with the person's "deepest personal beliefs can create other internal environments that can help the individual reach enhanced states of health and well-being." This combination of techniques is what Dr. Benson calls the "faith factor."

During my bout with cancer, meditation became an important part of my recovery. I experimented with many forms of meditation, becoming rather eclectic about methods. I combined the abdominal breathing and progressive relaxation and, becoming aware of my breathing, then repeated my phrase or word on which I focused as I exhaled. I found this particularly helpful in falling asleep at night when my mind was filled with disturbing thoughts that kept me awake, while waiting for surgery, sweating out test results, lying in a hospital bed, or just on a lovely day to enhance the beauty around me.

I also discovered that, as I walked or jogged, I could meditate using my focusing words or phrases in rhythm with my breathing in and out. I do this often when I finish my imagery and prayer time and still have a few miles to cover. Dr. Benson explains that while walking, you can't close your eyes as is required for the standard relaxation response technique, but the results can be just as rewarding as you watch where you are going. I find phrases from the 23rd Psalm most effective and comforting, although there are bits from favorite hymns that fit in nicely with my walking cadence.

I have been called upon these past few years to give encouragement to other cancer patients. Some are old friends and others new acquaintances with whom I share a bond. Hardly any of these people know what meditation is truly about and they still seem to associate it only with the Eastern mystical rites of transcendental meditation as used by Tibetan Buddhists. This was surprising to me, as so much is written today about meditation, and its healing benefits. I particularly like Joan Borysenko's definition of meditation which is "any activity that keeps the attention pleasantly anchored in the present moment."

Over the last few years there have been many approaches to the subject of disease linked to personality and unresolved problems. The Simontons believe that "our emotional and mental states play a significant role in both susceptibility to disease, including cancer, and in recovery from all disease." Bernie Siegel said of the outlook of Lawrence LeShan, noted psychologist and author, "Lack of emotional outlet is a common theme in histories of cancer patients." This might explain why cancer is more prevalent in convents than in prisons, where frustrations can be acted out more acceptably.

Despair and depression play havoc with our immune system. This has been demonstrated in many ways, and I believe that this is one reason why a few years ago many patients with AIDS did not want to receive their diagnoses and postponed having the HIV test. Once the diagnosis was given and there was no cure, the depression over a fatal diagnosis gave way to loss of hope and subsequent devastation of the immune system, as well as many suicides. Again, from the Simontons, "In the face of uncertainty there is nothing wrong with hope," but in the case of AIDS during the 1980s, there was never any hope given. I am not in complete agreement with all theories of the typical cancer patients' personalities, particularly the theories that implicate an unhappy childhood, lack of unconditional love, and feelings of unworthiness that may come and go through life.

According to the Simontons, these typical cancer patients are often "compulsively proper and generous people, who put the needs of others before their own." Ultimately, by continuing these routes, depleted and exhausted, supposedly this is when cancer can make its way into their bodies. While I can see many characteristics in those cancer patients whom I have known and also in myself, I think that self-blame is destructive and not a productive way to deal with survival.

These are all retrospective examinations of past events used to justify an illness. Nevertheless, if any other events that are still present during the course of cancer can be drastically changed, I believe that these changes could very well alter the course of the illness.

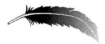

Making Positive
Life Changes

To illustrate how changing some unpleasant aspects of a person's life may sway the course of illness, I have a story about my friend Claudette, who developed breast cancer not too long after my ovarian cancer was treated.

Claudette did quite well for several years and then had a recurrence in her liver, which was discovered during her follow-up tests, although she felt very well and had no symptoms. Her first thought was to begin chemotherapy as soon as possible, as her oncologist had suggested, but Claudette had some reservations, as she was not satisfied with the attention she had been receiving. Claudette asked me if I could recommend another oncologist in Boston, which I did. She made an appointment.

She accepted the offer that Russ and I made to drive her to Boston, and we were amazed when she said that her husband didn't wish to go along with her. This was the first inkling that all was not well with her marriage.

As we rode to Boston carrying scan reports and other records, Claudette was most hopeful and eager to see this well-known surgical oncologist and envisioned being given a powerful, new type of chemotherapy that would cure her liver cancer.

I tried to be optimistic without giving false hope. I looked over the scans, both the new ones and those of several years back, and in comparing them told her that I couldn't see that they looked much different. Perhaps the suspicious areas were only cysts that had been there for ages. Certainly I was no expert, but I thought that strange things have been known to occur, and if I could keep her spirits up, what harm could it do?

Dr. C. read Claudette's records and examined her. Claudette then requested that Russ and I be with her during the consultation in the physician's office. Dr. C. asked Claudette how she felt and she told him, "Wonderful—better than I've felt in ages." Dr. C. questioned her about her children and other interests in her life. He said that he was "not impressed by the liver scans." He told her that he was not interested in doing tests, but was judging her on how she looked and how she felt.

In a gentle way, Dr. C. told Claudette that while others might not agree, his philosophy was, "If you feel well, why should I give you treatment that will make you sick and miserable, when the outcome will be the same?" He explained that she might opt to return to her local oncologist and have chemotherapy, or "go home and have a good summer with your kids."

When Claudette asked Dr. C., "Do I have liver cancer?" he answered her in such a way that he didn't say yes, but he didn't say no. This was all extremely thought provoking and came as a bitter blow to her.

I accompanied her to the ladies' room, not having any idea how I would handle this, and quickly said a prayer, asking that I might say the right things. Her first words were that she felt sick to her stomach and was going to vomit. "He told me I was going to die, didn't he?" she cried. I tried to clarify to Claudette my interpretation of what Dr. C. had told us, as she attempted to regain her bearings enough to leave and get out into fresh air. During the trip home, Claudette had pretty much made up her mind to enjoy the summer with her children, visit her mother, and get on with living.

There are many philosophies involved and decisions to make regarding cancer treatment, particularly when recurrence is a consideration. Apparently her unhappy marriage was one of the aspects of her life that she could change.

Claudette had read Dr. Bernie Siegel's book *Love, Medicine and Miracles* and we had shared our feelings of hope and ways of coping and maintaining a positive attitude, such as by meditation, during a life-threatening illness. She decided to go forward and make some positive and drastic changes in her life, which indeed took much courage.

This courageous young woman divorced her husband, moved out of her home, and continued at her job, which she loved and from which she received much satisfaction and support. She subsequently met and became involved in a loving relationship with a man who ultimately was there for her during the final stages of her illness.

By accepting the advice of Dr. C., Claudette enjoyed life immensely for several years in her new home, lifestyle, and relationship without medical therapy. Later, when bone metastasis developed, she was treated with radiation which relieved her pain and allowed her to keep working.

During this time, Claudette continued her meditation and imagery. Although she did not recover, she put up a monumental fight and lived her last few years to the fullest.

I feel certain that changing what she could of the unpleasant aspects of her life and participating in her own care—gaining control by making these decisions—was a positive choice for Claudette, particularly when we consider what treatments we endure, hoping for more time, rather than for the quality of what time we have left on this earth.

Misery

On Being Wretched

The human body can endure great physical assault, particularly when there is hope for healing.

From the time following my surgery and throughout the seven months of chemotherapy, even though I continued my self-healing practices, life wasn't exactly a bed of roses for many reasons. First of all, due to the extensive pelvic surgery that had been necessary to remove all the cancer, I had no feelings of having to urinate. I was not what you would consider incontinent, but I had to learn to time myself according to the amount of liquids that I had drunk and then use my abdominal muscles to start the voiding process.

This condition has remained and is similar to what is known as a neurogenic bladder. This is a dysfunction, often resulting when the local nerve supply to the urinary bladder and its outlet is disrupted. I understand that this is not uncommon following radical pelvic surgery. With today's new products on the market, you can easily find padding to meet individual needs. I have adapted quite well, although I doubt I could handle an African safari or a camel trek through Egypt.

The second problem that arose after surgery and during chemotherapy was an extremely tormenting bowel dysfunction. I attributed this to the effect of chemotherapy and fully expected my intestinal tract to return to its former function after the first year or so, but it did not. I felt as if I had a severe irritable colon. I constantly experienced the feeling of having a heavy weight low inside my abdomen pressing on my recto-sigmoid area.

Tests and exams showed nothing significant enough to cause such discomfort. I became a veritable bowel invalid and lived in fear of going anywhere, except for a few hours at a time. My nights were dreadful and the times after meals were very threatening to me. This continued—my fear of being away from home. The bathroom became my library, where I kept books, magazines, and newspapers. The time I spent there can be measured by the fact that I could complete the *New York Times* crossword puzzle in twenty-four hours.

Ernest Hemingway said, "Now is no time to think of what you do not have. Think of what you can do with what there is." I had my life, my mind, my senses, my arms and legs, and I used them.

When on my own turf, I did well. As a matter of fact, I was rather proud of myself that I could jog five miles a day, or go cross-country skiing, and probably had more stamina and agility than many other women I knew. But put me in a situation where I had to function socially, and I was a wreck. I was unable to make commitments, so I gave up committees and meetings and avoided any type of appointments whenever possible. Entertaining also threw me for a loop, because of my need to live day to day.

Planning ahead devastated me. Other than small family get-togethers, the only really enjoyable and unstressful type of entertaining I did was in the summer. On a warm, sunny day I could call friends for an impromptu swim in our pool and a cookout. These occasions always turned into happy times and made me feel human again.

As for other events that required planning, I didn't do very much and am sure that many of our more casual acquaintances probably didn't understand. After all, discussing your bowel problems is probably not high on the list of appropriate social discourse.

Even today, after all that I endured in attempts to cure my physical problem, this lifestyle of limited social interaction remains, but it is a small price to pay for my life.

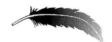

Rising Doubts

Litigation?

During my three-week hospitalization following the initial debulking surgery, Dr. A., the gynecologist who had been caring for me for about seven years, visited me daily, even on weekends. He was the one who did not detect my malignancy, and was no longer my physician. Dr. A. talked about his family and how he had spent his weekends. I enjoyed his visits. For well over a year he phoned me at fairly regular intervals to inquire how I was doing. On one occasion, he even called me from the airport to find out my state of health.

For some time I appreciated his thoughtfulness and was touched by his concern. I believed that he was sincere and probably remorseful that he had failed to diagnose my cancer. As time passed and I began reviewing the events pertaining to my illness, doubts began to bore their way into my mind. I wondered if I was a victim of negligence. I soon found that I wasn't the only one with suspicions; other family members and friends had apparently considered this from the beginning, but allowed me to come to this ponderous supposition on my own.

Did Dr. A. visit me because he was genuinely solicitous and interested in my well-being? Did he phone me often because he worried about his former patient? Or did he wonder if I was still alive? Could he have been afraid that I might blame him for failing to diagnose my cancer and seek legal action? Did he think it prudent to keep tabs on me?

My mistrust began to grow and hostility and bitterness toward Dr. A. brewed until I became so consumed with anger that I knew I could neither be at ease in my mind nor heal until I found out the answers.

> "And ye shall know the truth and the truth
> will make you free."
> —John 8:32

After much soul-searching Russ and I, with the full support and help of family and caring friends, began our quest for the "best" lawyer in Boston for handling medical malpractice litigation. We were successful in finding an outstanding attorney.

All pertinent material had been received by the lawyer prior to our first appointment, so he had familiarized himself with my case. He told us that because my prognosis was considered favorable and, due to the difficulty in diagnosing ovarian cancer, he could not be certain of the outcome of this type of case. He explained that it was his policy not to accept a case unless he knew for certain that he could win if it went to trial. He did, however, suggest that I would have no difficulty finding a lawyer who would be most willing to pursue this. We decided not to pursue this any further. In retrospect, I believe we made the right decision.

While I regret that Dr. A. failed me by not following

through with aggressive diagnostic techniques regardless of the benign-appearing report from the ultrasound procedures, I am not sure that my outcome could be any better. I do know that I would have had treatment four months earlier, therefore lessening much pain and deterioration of my general health and perhaps sparing me such devastating effects to my G.I. and urinary systems, which are permanent and adversely affect many parts of my life.

My purpose in writing about this episode is to explain that my decision to institute a lawsuit against Dr. A., the preparations, research, and the actual appointment and consultation with the lawyer, served as a means of venting my anger—somewhat like writing a nasty letter to someone but never mailing it. Knowing more, as I do today, about the complexities involved in the diagnosis of ovarian cancer, I would not recommend to those afflicted with this disease that they attempt litigation based *only* on failure to diagnose.

This situation has taken me many years to resolve, but has been a valuable measure in the closure process. I believe I can now let this part of my life rest in peace. Even though I can't say that I found the "truth," I did seek it to my satisfaction.

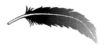

The G.I. Episode

Early in the spring of 1991 Dr. Barton referred me to a highly respected gastroenterologist. My symptoms were so diverse that I always found myself at a loss in describing them. When I found this to be so during my first appointment, my new doctor asked me how I felt at the moment as I was sitting in his office. I said, "I feel as if I had a twenty-pound bag of cement inside my lower G.I. tract thumping around and trying to push through a straw."

I went through countless tests. There were laboratory studies and a lactose tolerance test. A sigmoidoscopy was done and I had a consultation with a nutritionist. I tried a few medications that offered no relief and I was instructed to keep a daily diary of my G.I. functions. Living it was bad enough, but writing about it was not easy for me. This journal was presented to the doctor at each appointment and I was to phone him about every two weeks to report on my condition or discuss the effectiveness of the medications.

As kind and esteemed as this doctor was, I somehow had a feeling that he didn't really hear me, that he never really understood the pain I was enduring. I still had no diagnosis and no relief. Perhaps I had him baffled.

On my final visit that fall, he told me that a low sigmoid colostomy would give me the relief that I deserved. Being so miserable and vulnerable, I was grateful that finally help was available. At this point, I would have gone along with anything suggested that would provide relief. After conferring with Dr. Barton, we both agreed, as did Russ, that this procedure sounded like the solution to my problems, and I was eager to get on with it.

A colostomy is a surgically created artificial opening from the colon to the outside of the body. This allows intestinal contents to pass through into a pouch attached by some type of adhesive to the abdomen. The exposed portion of the intestine around which the pouch is applied is called a stoma.

The surgery was performed by Dr. Barton at the New England Baptist Hospital in October 1991, and herein lies another tale of survival.

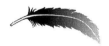

Flashbacks

This tale has disturbing memories, but reminds me, on occasions when I feel like a wimp, that I can be tough when I need to be.

During these years, I had many episodes of flashbacks, particularly related to odors reminiscent of my initial surgery and especially of the chemotherapy. Each time it became necessary to return to the hospital, fears returned that I thought I had worked through and put behind me. I found this was not so. I thought that my hospitalization for the colostomy would not be overly disturbing, but I underestimated the power of the body's ability to recall odors from the past.

I remember so well that, during my seven months of chemotherapy and for another two or three years, I kept my small purple cosmetic case well hidden in the back of my bathroom closet so I wouldn't have to look at it when I opened the door. This is the case that accompanied me to the hospital when I had my surgery and chemotherapy treatments. One glance at this innocent-seeming case evoked such strong memories that I became nauseated to the point of vomiting.

Of all our senses, smell is supposedly the one most linked to memory. I discovered this to be true for me on several occasions when various olfactory exposures retrieved unpleasant experiences related to my illness. This was very unnerving. Walking along the freshly washed and waxed floors of the New England Baptist Hospital headed for a routine appointment, I noticed an odor that I couldn't immediately identify. After a few seconds of nausea and anxiety, I recognized the scent of the same cleaning substance used daily by the person who cleaned the floor in my room when I had been a patient many times for surgeries and chemotherapy.

Another example of what I call olfactory flashbacks occurred while visiting a relative in another hospital several years after my treatments ended. In taking a wrong turn to reach our destination, we passed through the oncology unit. Although no one else detected any unusual odor, it was unmistakably the revolting smell of "chemo" that found its way straight to the pit of my stomach.

This odor, unidentifiable to those who have not had to endure chemotherapy and its associated horrors, permeated not only my nose, but my whole body, as well. After our visit, I rode in the car with the window wide open, breathing in the cold December air, unable to rid myself of this smell for many miles.

So now I was back at the Baptist again for a colostomy, not anticipating any formidable events. I wasn't thrilled to be having this procedure, but I accepted it as necessary to improve the quality of my life. Then the unexpected happened. The odor of the bed linen and towels nearly drove me out of my mind. I asked my husband, to bring in my favorite room spray, my very special cologne, and even, as a last resort, Vicks VapoRub to put in my nostrils. Nothing helped!

Everyone reassured me that there was no unpleasant odor in anything with which I came in contact, yet the feelings of panic that accompanied these flashbacks persisted. I was reliving the feeling of the cool bed as I pulled the sheet and cotton blanket over me waiting for the IV nurse to start my chemotherapy, dreading what was ahead.

I told Dr. Barton, "I've got to get out of here!" He told me that as soon as I could care for my colostomy, I would be discharged. With that news, I became a fast learner. By the next morning I had become an "expert" and was on my way home.

One more rugged ordeal behind me, and I survived it!

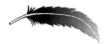

Living with a Colostomy

My Comedy of Errors

Before I begin the account of my adventures with my colostomy, let me explain that I tried very hard to deal with this "outside plumbing" with as much humor as I could muster—sometimes joking and fighting back tears at the same time.

Norman Cousins in his book *Head First, the Biology of Hope* entitles one whole chapter "The Laughter Connection." Among his conclusions from his research is that laughter can be a powerful painkiller, probably by activating the release of endorphins, which are the body's natural painkillers and actually increase the number of disease-fighting immune cells.

Cousins also quotes from a report on research by Dr. James Walsh, over half a century ago, detailing the "beneficial effects of laughter on the lungs, liver, heart, pancreas, spleen, stomach, intestines and brain." He wrote that "laughter has the effect of brushing aside many of the worries and fears that set the stage for sickness."

I have noticed that over the past few years my sense of humor has changed. Things that I would have considered to be in poor taste I must say find me chuckling inside, because I say to myself, "Anything for a good laugh, if not at the expense of anyone else." Nurses have always been noted for a particularly strange sense of humor, which many consider inappropriate, just to allow us to survive critical events and morbid scenes.

Some ovarian cancer patients come out of surgery with ostomies. Some are permanent, some are temporary, depending upon what had to be removed in the debulking process to get rid of all tumor. While this did not happen to me, when the need for a colostomy arose later, neither Dr. Barton nor I had any reason to believe that it was not to be permanent. Although it was a Hartmann procedure, leaving the rectum intact so that reconnection was possible, it was neither a probability nor even a consideration at the time. So what I relate, regarding my experiences living with a colostomy, does not in any way impart the impression that I took it lightly, or believed that it was only temporary and something to deal with for a short time. This was for real—another challenge.

I was truly "into it." From the beginning, I decided that it was to be no secret that I had a colostomy and I never tried to hide the fact that "it" was a part of me, although I never stood up and shouted. I was very fortunate, from the beginning when I came home, to have Jerra Sullivan, an enterostomal therapist, who came to the house and started me off in the right direction.

Without Jerra I don't know what I would have done, because coming home from the hospital with a colostomy was like coming home with a new baby. It kept me up all night, it demanded the same sort of cleanups, and it took up just about all of my time. The only difference was it never did get to the point where it would sleep through the night.

As time progressed, the only change I noticed in my bowel function was that instead of functioning through the normal channels, it functioned through the stoma. In other words, instead of spending my time sitting doing crossword puzzles, I spent the time kneeling on my gardening cushion on the bathroom floor emptying my pouch.

Ethel Barrymore once said, "When life knocks you to your knees—well, that's the best position to pray, isn't it?"

I was delighted, however, to find that the technology in ostomy care had greatly improved since my nursing days. Gone are the old smelly rubbery equipment and the various cements, and the terrible outlook given to patients who had ostomies back in the fifties. I used to think during my nursing days that if I were to have an ostomy, it would have to be one of the worst things that could ever happen to me. I now know there are many things that can happen to alter a life much more than having an ostomy.

I regularly received a newsletter from the company whose ostomy products I used. In it there was a great exchange of ideas and helpful suggestions from others who were living with ostomies. Many who had ostomies had them for reasons different from mine. A great majority of correspondents had lived with inflammatory bowel disease for so long that to them having an ileostomy was the most wonderful thing that could have happened. It gave them a whole new lease on life, coming as a blessed relief. I also found that a lot of people with colostomies had had them for many years. A great proportion of them were men, and they seemed to handle things far better than I was able to do.

I learned the hard way that what sounded like an efficient method of caring for an ostomy doesn't always work in practice, particularly for women. One source of information, for example, describes the simplicity of draining a pouch in a public rest room. For a man who can easily lean over a urinal and carries his wet wipes with him, I am sure that the procedure could be handled quite well.

I was never able to succeed in a public rest room. Being inexperienced in this new lifestyle, but priding myself on being an innovative nurse, I carried equipment wherever I went. No matter what I was told, I found that there was no way to drain my pouch without being down on my knees, which is not easy when you are enclosed in a booth with people on both sides of you. There you are, down on the hard, dirty floor—never knowing when a curious toddler's face would peer up at you from the adjoining stall.

Even with all the helpful hints and advice from the experts, unpalatable as this may be, splashing and odor were inevitable. Caring for my colostomy away from home was not a good experience. Nothing I had read mentioned how to handle the clothing situation with skirts or dresses and panty hose being in the way. Wearing slacks simplified the procedure somewhat, but even then there was the possibility of a sweater or blouse dropping down over your strategic area of operation. I kept clothespins and hair clips with me to help hold up my clothing, should the need arise, and then I would attempt this procedure only if I were in an area that offered privacy.

I had a dreadful experience one of the few times that the necessity arose to drain away from home. One of the clips let go, my sweater dropped, and, to add fuel to the fire, I had left my bifocals at home. I shed tears over this one, as I felt like a total failure. I was also mad as hell!

Dostoyevski wrote that "man is a pliable animal—a being who gets accustomed to everything." Perhaps this is so, but this woman just wasn't very pliable. I preferred to stay close to home instead of risking a catastrophe, particularly after a meal. There were some events, however, where my presence was necessary. Needless to say, I was not at ease.

I discovered that my stoma could emit rather loud and strange noises with no warning whatsoever: particularly unnerving while walking through a buffet line when both hands were busy. I was told that pressing my arm or hand firmly over the ostomy would muffle the noise, but I was always too late.

Following an afternoon of league bowling in the noisy alley and feeling quite complacent, as all was quiet on my "home front," I went to the mall to browse through one of the large department stores. The store was nearly deserted and extremely quiet as I looked through a rack of blouses. A clerk appeared and asked if she might help me.

I looked up at her and as our eyes met, my ostomy let go with a loud blast, starting as a high-pitched whistle and coming down the scale to a low note on a tuba. Her eyes grew wide as she looked at me, bewildered. In a state of shock I made the quick decision that I owed her no explanations, so I said, "No thank you, I was looking for a lime green blouse," and with that I turned slowly and dawdled deliberately along to the door.

Reaching the exit, I made fast tracks to the car and thought, "I can let this thing destroy me and have a good bawl for myself, or have a much needed laugh for the relief that I need"—and laugh I did. I also repeated this story many times—not very *polite* humor, but this is the way I handled it.

I learned from this experience to carry my purse over my left arm and press it snugly against me when in a quiet area. Many times I dined in fine restaurants hugging tightly to my left side for dear life. Dinner music in the background always gave me a feeling of relaxation in more ways than you could imagine.

I am blessed with a husband who has shared with me a marriage that has endured the vow "for better or worse." Russ has been my soul mate and my support unselfishly throughout these twelve very difficult years. When I was diagnosed with ovarian cancer, he and my family were devastated. However, when Russ saw that I intended to fight and was determined to be around for a long time, I think that he, too, was very encouraged and joined in my fight to survive and to enjoy our life together, the best we could. Many changes had to be made.

For these twelve years, the especially challenging ones, he gave above and beyond what was expected of him. When I had the colostomy, I don't think he had any idea of what to expect, what it looked like, the care it involved, and the changes it would bring about in our marriage. However, after he first took a good look at my stoma, the round, pink "rosebud" at the end of my bowel that protruded out of the left side of my abdomen, he befriended it and shared in its care. As we went to the medical supply store for the first time, the clerk waiting on us said, "I really couldn't tell which one of you had the colostomy."

While I took complete day-to-day and night-to-night care of this thing that I call "outside plumbing," the one thing Russ determined he could do better than I was to fit and apply my disk or wafer. The wafer has an adhesive backing and must fit perfectly around the stoma and stick securely to the skin. The pouch then snaps into a ring on the wafer. This he did with his engineering expertise and loving hands, which very few men could have or would have done, at least from what I have heard and read. He still has the last piece, the little round paper that backs the disk, from the very last application before I finally was reconnected in the hospital. Stuck in the mirror on his bureau is the little round disk with a smile that he drew on it.

Nightmares—One and Two

Another Trial, Another Triumph

In the spring of 1993, it was becoming increasingly evident that the colostomy was not the answer to my G.I. problems. Dr. Barton referred me to Dr. Ronald Bleday, an excellent colon-rectal surgeon at another Boston hospital for evaluation and testing to determine if reconnecting my bowel and eliminating the colostomy was feasible. The tests included barium enemas and something called a defecography. This last test I will not elaborate upon except to say that it is a humbling experience; however, the staff was most professional and allowed me to retain a certain amount of dignity. I appreciated their kindness.

After receiving the news that I was a good candidate for having my colostomy put back, a date was set for the surgery. In July I entered the hospital and had the surgery. During the procedure, a very unusual condition was found and I describe this because I think it is important clinically. There are unusual anatomical changes that can develop following radical debulking surgery for ovarian cancer, such as what was done to me to save my life, that long-term survivors can present. Intestinal dysfunctions are apparently common and may develop early after surgery. My problem may have been progressing for years, culminating in this course of events.

A rectal loop had formed between my sacrum and rectum, which was one of the areas where a large mass of tumor had been removed. Over a period of time, this loop became fixed in with scar tissue, and new blood vessels had grown around it. During the surgery to put back my colostomy, Dr. Bleday discovered this and changed the procedure in order to repair it. He removed this loop and joined the remaining ends together, the anastamosis, or surgical connection, being only about two and a half inches above the anus. Technically, this procedure was described as a partial colectomy with coloproctostomy, low pelvic anastamosis with colostomy. The temporary double-barreled colostomy would allow healing to occur. This unexpected surgical procedure took about seven hours.

The plan was to wait a few months for healing and then complete the process of reconnecting my intestine, ultimately leaving me without a colostomy. Apparently this phenomenon had not been seen before, and did not show up in any of the many examinations I had. A loop in the recto-sigmoid area often appears and shows up in X-rays of the lower G.I. tract, but the loop is freely movable and changes into a normal position. There was apparently no way to know that, in my case, the loop was fixed; only during this type of surgery could it have been discovered. Following the surgical procedure, Dr. Bleday said that, in reexamining my various X-rays and, even knowing what he then knew, he found no such problem detectable from the radiological information.

From my experience as a long-term survivor of ovarian cancer, I would conclude that there are many conditions that can develop following extensive debulking surgery, some of which have perhaps never before been encountered. I would, therefore, recommend to those women who are experiencing severe gastrointestinal difficulties to request a thorough G.I. examination to rule out or to discover any condition similar to mine.

Recovery from this surgery was extremely stressful. I was in a different environment from that of the New England Baptist Hospital, where I had received such loving care throughout my three previous operations and all of my chemotherapy. Due to the unforeseen nature of the operation and the time required to accomplish this procedure, as well as the positioning on the operating table, there was apparently pressure on various nerves. This resulted in many painful and debilitating obstacles to recovery.

As soon as I awakened in the recovery room, I was first aware of such leg pain that I said to the nurse, "Oh my God, I must have had another hamstring tear!" This was pain I had known before. She told me that it was from trauma to my sciatic nerve, a result of the long surgical procedure.

Medication kept me sedated and the pain under control for a day or so; consequently, I was unaware of the weakness in my right leg or of the paresthesias (abnormal sensations) I had. I gradually became aware of the numbness in my right leg. I had no feeling from my knee to my ankle and very diminished feeling, actually numbness, in my inner thigh and groin extending to my lower buttock and peri-anal area. Being on medication kept me from experiencing any severe pain while I was hospitalized. It waited until I went home.

The first awareness of the severity of this new disability came when I was allowed to get out of bed. My leg just buckled beneath me and I realized that I could not stand, to say nothing of walking to a chair.

After a few of my many tubes were removed, and with the help of a fine and caring physical therapist, I learned to use a walker and eventually progressed to a cane and managing stairs. I was still unable to get out of bed by myself. This hampered my convalescence, as I valued my self-reliance whenever possible and particularly because the nursing care wasn't up to my standards.

I had been aware ahead of time through Boston newspapers and television that much of the direct patient care at this hospital was provided by nursing aides, many of whom had very limited training and experience. However, I was not prepared for the severity of the situation I encountered following my surgery, which lasted until I was discharged.

Lying in bed, I was absolutely helpless amid tubes, lines, pumps, and pouches. I had a central line for administration of fluids and medications. This tubing is attached to an indwelling catheter that is surgically placed into a large central vein in the neck. This line is attached to an infusion pump.

I had a little gadget that I could press, which would release morphine to ease my pain. This is called a PCA, or patient-controlled analgesia. A nasogastric tube drained stomach fluids into another pump. Placed in my abdominal incision was a tube attached to a plastic container called a Jackson-Pratt pump, which stayed with me in bed. Having just unexpectedly acquired a new colostomy, I had a large pouch attached to my left side. From my bladder, a catheter and tubing drained into a bag hanging under the bed. My legs were encased in some sort of pressure-gradient stockings to increase the deep venous blood circulation and prevent thrombosis.

The nurses were very adept and professional in tending to all of my appliances and "machinery," but, as to any hands-on care, I found it greatly lacking. Somewhere between the first and second day, I pleaded for the chance to wash my hands and brush my teeth, or at least to rinse my mouth. Discovering that it would take an act of Congress, I gave up. Eventually I did have some slight exposure to something cool and damp—I was given a wet facecloth!

Two frail young aides felt sure they could get me on my feet and assist me to a chair. My warnings regarding my right leg buckling like a piece of rubber hose seemed to be disregarded, so I refused to get out of bed until two men were available to lift me to my chair. The last thing I needed was a fractured hip!

It was during these episodes that I realized that most of these aides knew very little or nothing about the origin or insertion of my tubes. I tried to keep them from being dislodged when I was moved and gotten up, but a few were stepped on now and then in the moving process. Thankfully, Russ was there to intervene before the tubes were accidentally yanked out.

On the second or third day, when I was given the chance to bathe myself, about 8 a.m., I made a special request that I be moved to my chair and given my tub of water early because Russ, who came daily, was bringing our daughter Nancy late in the morning when visiting hours began. Suffice it to say, at noon I was still in the chair, covered in a towel, with an unmade bed.

To add a bit of humor to this situation, the bath "ritual" was incredible. The items I needed from my bedside table couldn't be found by the aide. Then, one by one, she would locate the various articles—soap, toothbrush, towels, lotion. When I requested powder, she found my lovely talcum and shook it all over the tub of water. Unbelievable—but true!

I did have a heartwarming experience that I treasure. On one of my worst nights, my body and spirit wretched, I lay in bed like a beached whale, soaked with perspiration. Somewhere after midnight, in response to my light, a young, smiling chubby lady in a pink uniform appeared and said, "Honey, I'm going to fix you all up comfy," and she did.

This dear soul bathed me, rubbed my back, changed my linens, and brought several soft pillows, which she positioned in just the right areas. Then she brought another soft, small pillow and gave it to me to "hug like a teddy bear."

I watched for her the next few nights but she never came back. I later learned that she had been sent from another floor to help out for a few hours. I know that I have a guardian angel and that my friend in pink was sent to me that night on a rescue mission.

A highlight of this hospital stay: Although I was not at the New England Baptist Hospital, and not Dr. Barton's patient for this particular surgery, he and Nancy Bray visited me "unofficially" every day.

The neurology department was consulted to assess the nerve injuries that occurred during surgery. Prior to the visit by the neurologist, one young aspiring doctor, whose status in the hierarchy I don't recall, bounded into my room in his running shoes, introduced himself, and threw his backpack onto a chair. He proceeded to conduct a neurological examination on me in a quite thorough and professional manner.

Halfway through the exam, in response to one of his questions, I answered with a descriptive phrase common to those of us with a medical background. "How do you know those terms?" he asked me, temporarily distracted. "Do you have some type of medical background?"

I replied that I was a registered nurse and that these anatomical terms were second nature to me. Quickly, he reached for my chart, thumbed through it, and said, "There's nothing in your record stating that you are an R.N."

"Probably not," I replied. "Should there be?"

He said, "If it had been on your chart that you were an R.N., you would have received the VIP treatment."

Under my breath, I quickly said to myself, "I sure could use it." Then, regrouping my thoughts, I found these implications most interesting. This man continued to be very professional, but he began to let his guard down somewhat and relate to me on a collegial level, smiled, and seemed more friendly.

This was a week of many dark hours in my fight for survival. The fortunate discovery and repair of the loop of bowel by Dr. Bleday was joyous news. I wasn't thrilled to be going home with another colostomy, but the reason for it counteracted the blow. What I suffered during this hospitalization was another notch on my survival stick. I also learned that I needed to be more assertive, but before anyone wonders why I put up with such poor care, remember—I knew that I had to go back! I had decided that, on returning to have my surgical procedure completed, I would not let this situation repeat itself. When I was safely home, I would handle things in a propitious way.

After my discharge, I spent the remainder of the summer walking gingerly with a cane, having gotten beyond the need for a walker. Going up and down the stairs wasn't too bad, as long as I remembered which leg started up first and then reversing when I headed down. Speaking of heading—I only took two "headers," both going downstairs.

During this summer of 1993 my leg strengthened gradually and the sciatic pain decreased. The paresthesias and abnormal nerve sensations remained and were extremely painful, particularly in my buttock, groin, and inner thigh area, making many routine activities nearly impossible. I could not tolerate even the slightest pressure from underclothing or my necessary padding. I fashioned all sorts of strange-looking devices from flannel and fleece that I tried to use as a barrier between my skin and clothing, but discovered that nerve pain is not easily assuaged.

Out of desperation, I had about five acupuncture treatments, which I believe relieved the sciatica but did very little to ease the burning pain in my thigh area. With time, the acute pain diminished but now, after nearly five years, there are still paresthesias that cause much physical and emotional discomfort.

I had hoped the remaining nerve damage would eventually heal, but so far there has been no improvement. This branch of the small sciatic nerve affects part of my buttock and the right half of my perineal (crotch) area. This affliction is a real "pain in the butt" and is causing many more challenges in my already changed lifestyle.

Sitting for any length of time can be unbearable. Traveling any great distance aggravates the condition and leaves me extremely sore for several days, even when I use a special cushion. My beautiful beach bicycle with its custom padded seat is gathering dust in the basement. I bought it when I was unable to jog due to a stress fracture in my foot. I was still able to pedal, though, and rode many miles along the beach roads blending my imagery and meditation with the sounds and smells of the ocean. The sensation of sitting on sharp burning needles now makes cycling impossible.

This anecdote has an ironic twist. This nerve injury is the result of the only surgical procedure I anticipated with joy. I was on top of the world about to be rid of my colostomy. I dreamed about it but never thought it would be possible. I did lose my colostomy—but I lost another part of myself as well.

I have discovered that there is a price to be paid for winning. While I don't like the various discomforts and inconveniences, the alternative would be worse. I try to conquer the bitterness and anger over this painful nerve trauma I must live with by the knowledge that such an attitude is spiritually and physically destructive. I don't always succeed.

I was hopeful that I would be ready for my final surgery in four to six weeks. I had been told to eat well and build myself up. I had two low barium enemas to determine when healing was complete. These exams showed that the healing was slower than anticipated, so surgery was delayed.

When I returned to the same hospital in November, I was really "built up" to the tune of ten pounds gained from a lot of good food and no exercise, but I was ready. Although I was most eager to be rid of my colostomy and put this exhaustive series of events behind me, I entered the hospital with much apprehension after the previous ordeal.

Russ and I left for Boston early in the morning, my preparation being completed at home the previous day. Naturally, I was very empty and hungry and feeling dehydrated. On arrival, we discovered that my 9:30 a.m. surgery had been postponed due to an emergency. The phone call advising me of this change in schedule apparently came too late, since we departed from home about 5 a.m.

We walked up and down the halls of the hospital's main floor, smelling the coffee, and sat in various waiting rooms, watching the clock as the minutes and hours dragged by unmercifully. I finally reached the point where it seemed best to say good-bye to Russ and be admitted to the operating room "holding" area. I felt like I was in an airport where the sign read, ONLY TICKETED PASSENGERS BEYOND THIS POINT.

During the O.R. admission routine, I told the physician, who I think was an anesthesiologist, that, due to my bowel prep and lack of fluids, my electrolytes were "out of whack." Since 1986, I knew quite well to listen to my body. I usually know when my potassium is too low because muscles in my legs begin to twitch, leading to cramping.

I mentioned that I had had problems with electrolytes during the previous surgery and perhaps they could be averted by IV therapy started early. I don't know whether or not he listened to me or gave me much credibility because my routine IV was not started for some time, and I'm not at all sure what was added to it.

So there I was, after the admission procedure, lying beside other patients being prepared for various transplants, bypasses, and other surgeries. They were wheeled out to the O.R. while new patients were admitted, and I watched them leave also. But I just lingered, waiting on the gurney, unsedated, for several more hours. Once I seriously considered climbing down off the hard cart and leaving, taking my colostomy back home with me. Thaddeus told me it wasn't such a great idea. I had stuck a small yellow "smile" on my pouch to bid it a fond adieu. Whether anyone smiled when they removed my pouch for the last time, I'll never know. Not everybody shares my sense of humor.

Lying and waiting for so long was exhausting—both mentally and physically. I craved sleep, but was unable to doze off. The way that I survived this ordeal was by eliciting the relaxation response, meditating, and praying. The 23rd Psalm, always a comfort to me, gave me solace, as I repeated it over and over again. Finally, by midafternoon, my turn arrived. The surgery went quite well, with no unexpected events.

My stay in the recovery room was much longer than usual, due to a serious problem with my electrolytes. No one told me this, but I had the feeling that the staff feared I might go into cardiac arrest at any moment. Perhaps not, but I was aware of the problems that could develop when there are severe depletions of these electrolytes. After this crisis began to stabilize, I was moved to my room in a different building from where I was in July. For this I was most grateful!

The remainder of my stay was very pleasant and the nursing care was outstanding. I was cared for by nearly all R.N.s who were as kind and compassionate as they were skilled. My faith in the nursing profession was restored. As we became better acquainted, I told these nurses about some of the unbelievable episodes from my last admission. They were as appalled as I was.

My electrolytes were still low enough to cause my doctors to be concerned, even though I kept reiterating that this is a common happening whenever I lose copious amounts of fluid from my bowel during presurgical prep involving laxatives, enemas, or irrigations. I have learned to recognize this condition, of mild electrolyte imbalance, from previous bouts of diarrhea and from the great loss of fluid through my perspiration while jogging on a hot, humid day.

The electrolytes that were so low—sodium, potassium, and magnesium—finally reached normal enough levels, but Dr. Bleday thought that I should be evaluated by a nephrologist. I agreed and had a consultation and tests. This nephrologist told me that we might never truly know the cause of this enigma, but he considered it quite possible that cisplatin had caused some kidney damage, which was showing up only under stress.

He then asked me if I had been under much stress lately. I casually replied, "What about having Stage III C metastatic ovarian cancer, a colostomy, and two more major bowel surgeries?" I have never received a report from Dr. Bleday but, in all honesty, I didn't request it. I wasn't ready to open a can of worms, and felt confident that I knew my body quite well and the way it reacted under certain stresses.

Some may think that I have been too harsh in my censure of this hospital and my care. Some may also question whether I had a delayed bout of displaced or misplaced anger because I had ovarian cancer and was embittered by the delay in diagnosis. I think this is not the case. I believe my criticism is valid.

Dr. Gerald Epstein, a psychiatrist and a pioneer in waking dream therapy, says that it is not "wrong or bad" to feel anger, but it should be "managed," as should all emotions, both negative and positive. He suggests that we "acknowledge their presence and then deal with them."

I am dealing with the anger I felt by baring my soul, so to speak, in this story of surviving a deadly killer disease. My anger is directed at what I perceive as incompetency, and I believe this anger is justified.

Being human, we are all subject to making mistakes. I've certainly made my share. However, when we entrust ourselves into the safekeeping of those who are expected to be competent and for whose services we pay, we have the right to presume them worthy of our trust. We should expect those who are considered professionals in their fields to have the skills, knowledge, experience, and time to function in a competent manner where human lives are involved.

In the final operation to put back my colostomy, the top layer of my incision was left open to allow healing to occur from the inside and also to lessen the possibility of infection. After returning home, I had the visiting nurses twice daily for irrigations and dressings, gradually decreasing to only once a day. The area needing the care was in just the wrong spot for me to treat myself. After a few weeks, we taught Russ how to do the procedure and he lovingly and expertly took over my care. By Christmas Day I was healed. What a wonderful gift!

Another triumph—I survived!

About the time of my wound healing, another unexpected development occurred. My new intestinal system was not behaving properly and kept me busy night and day. Tests showed that I had contracted a mean "bug" known as Clostridium difficile.

C. difficile is something I wouldn't wish on anyone, but contracting the nasty organism is always a possibility when you are a hospital patient, and particularly when undergoing intestinal surgery. It is fairly common in nursing homes and easy to contract under certain circumstances. Infants and elderly people are particularly susceptible. This organism is often the cause of antibiotic- associated diarrhea, especially in people whose immune systems are compromised by disease or by chemotherapy. Ironically, the treatment consists of antibiotics, and relapse is not uncommon.

Of course, I did suffer a relapse, but the second course of treatment was successful and, again, I survived!

Ad Interim

Van, the Berkshires, Family, and Healing Places

During these last twelve years, although I may have given the impression that I had been a recluse due to my continuing intestinal problem, this was not so. There were many happy events that I enjoyed and that were very important to me, as well as other events where my presence was necessary. Whatever the occasion, it required planning ahead regarding my diet, liquid intake, and medication. By the time I left home, I had usually worked myself into such a snit that I was a nervous wreck.

Unfortunately, this situation still exists, but I am trying to work this out so that I don't perceive the situation as being so threatening. Since I must live this way, as part of the price I had to pay for my life, I realize that I must find a way to overcome my fear, particularly as I usually make it home without serious incident. Usually, but not always!

Early in 1987, I returned to some of my previous activities, such as attending University of New Hampshire hockey games and rejoining my bowling league, where I had been a member for more than twenty-five years. It was there that I made my first public appearance without my wig, showing off my tight ringlets. I remember how cold my head felt that winter, but how thrilled I was to have my own hair again.

When the snow arrived, Russ and I put on our cross-country skis and headed back through our woods, reblazing old trails for miles. It was awesome with the new heavy snow weighing down the hemlocks, the sun's radiance creating fields of glistening diamonds, as we glided on in glorious silence. The only signs of life, after a heavy snow in this wilderness, were the hoof-prints of the deer who had gone ahead of us. After wondering if I would live and ever again experience this sublime joy that I had so loved for years, I thanked God over and over for allowing me to be alive.

I felt the same gratitude when summer came and Russ and I returned for the first time to Odiorne's Point, only a few minutes from our home. We walked the path leading to the rocks that jut out to the ocean and sat, soaking in the sun and breathing in the salt air. Seagulls and cormorants soared and dove and rested on the rocks nearby. Ships passed out of the harbor while others returned to port.

I would find it difficult to choose among the grandeur of the sea, the beauty of the snow, and the majesty of the mountains, particularly during New England's foliage splendor. How very fortunate I am to have all these special places near our home in Portsmouth or our little house in the Berkshires. These particular places, as well as our first home, Key West, which we visit in the winter now that I am better able to travel a bit, are what I call my "healing places" because it is in these spots that I really feel the joy and importance of being alive.

Returning to the spring of 1987, we encountered a new problem. This difficult situation involved a beloved family member, Russ's dad, whom everyone called Van. Looking back, I know that our escapes involving him prove that God never gives us more than we can handle.

The tale of Van, my father-in-law, could be a story of its own, so I must restrict myself to the problems we encountered, how we dealt with them, and how they affected the physical problems related to my ovarian cancer. Without a sense of humor, Russ and I never could have survived those seven years and kept our sanity.

Van, once a brilliant engineer and inventor with numerous other talents, had a difficult time adjusting to the death of his wife, Russ's stepmother, whom we called Tom. She was adored by all of our family. Van became more and more of an unconventional free spirit and caused many a commotion in his area of the Berkshires. Having sold his farm in Cummington, Massachusetts, his home was now a small house in Dalton, Massachusetts, which had been nearer to his job as an engineer in Pittsfield before he retired.

Several years before the chaos began, he became angry and somewhat paranoid at the various utility companies, resulting in no longer having water, phone, or electricity. His house was not a safe place for him to stay, but it was home and no matter where we relocated him, he always went back to the only place he loved.

Van did not have Alzheimer's or any other diagnosed dementia; he was just a lovable, elderly man with many eccentricities. When the situation required our intervention, he was eighty-seven years old. The essence of this story is that he became unable to care for himself, according to societal standards, and we were forced to find a home where he could be supervised minimally, cared for and fed, yet maintain his mobility.

Van was very mobile! Only recently had he lost his car and driver's license, his moped, and finally his bicycle—all the result of various collisions. He was still a strong man, with strong legs, still proud of the fact that he had been on the Lehigh wrestling team and later the wrestling coach at Union College. He also knew how to ride a bus!

The Berkshire area was his home; even if we could have cared for him here in New Hampshire, he would not have been happy. But this was impossible for many reasons. First, it was a struggle for me to take care of myself, with Russ assuming many of our responsibilities. Both of us being only children, we had others who also needed our attention. Russ's mother, living alone about twenty five miles away from Van, was also having health problems. My mother, who lives near us, was quite healthy and a great help to me, but my illness had a strong effect on her and the worry took its toll in many ways. She developed Ménière's disease and later began having visual impairment, as well as other health problems.

So here we were in the spring of 1987, up to our necks in crazy situations, not exactly conducive to healing, yet somehow we managed. Perhaps it was just what I needed, although I didn't think so at the time.

We were obliged to make speed runs back and forth to western Massachusetts to handle some incredible situations. With my G.I. system in such a sorry state, being backed up on the Mass. Turnpike on a holiday weekend (unintentional) and feeling imminent diarrhea created an indescribable panic situation. This was just the beginning, and yet we managed. I survived to endure many more such tests of fortitude.

On one occasion, we were called to rescue Van after he had spent a night in the Berkshire County Jail for creating a commotion at his bank. Apparently he had heard that the bank was in trouble. He wanted to withdraw his money immediately and the process wasn't fast enough for him. He had grown increasingly distrustful of banks and various other establishments. In his impatience, he became agitated, and the bank officials called the police. The strange part of this story is that the bank did fold shortly after he had, with difficulty, closed out his account.

Early one winter, everything went from bad to worse. Van told us that an Asian waitress where he sometimes ate (we think on the house) offered to take care of him if he'd give her his house. We didn't pursue this or give it much credence, but later we did find her proposal in writing. Soon we became involved with one of the "helping" agencies, and an evaluation was conducted in the psychiatric unit of a large medical center. Because he could not be released without a place to go, he spent a very happy winter at this psychiatric unit in a lovely room, with fine food and care. This winter gave us the first peace of mind we had known in a long time. We knew Van was safe.

We felt fortunate to find a private home that had a few men living in a supervised setting with good home cooking and also on the bus route. Our Pittsfield lawyer had his father in the home and recommended it to us. We bought him new clothes, labeled them, and left feeling most relieved. Van was on the bus and back in his own house before we even reached the turnpike. This happened several times in other "nice" places we found for him. The phone would be ringing as we walked in the door, telling us, "Van left."

We found one home in an ideal rural setting near a favorite stop-over for Canada geese. Van stayed about an hour, then trudged along toward the highway. A state trooper picked him up and dropped him off in town. Van phoned us to say he left because he couldn't walk outside the door without stepping in "goose shit."

Russ and I were even sued for "elder abuse" because we couldn't keep him under control. Of course, this was not valid. We did our best. Eventually, after a few hospital-izations, one for much-needed prostate surgery, nursing home care was necessary. After being fortunate enough to find a bed for him, he rebelled. The chaos nearly ruined us, as well as Van and the staff. Ultimately, we placed him in a fine nursing home where he became resigned to the situa-tion and reverted to his lovable self. He spent his remain-ing years in this caring home and died in 1994 at the age of ninety-four.

While Van was at this nursing home in Lenox, we visit-ed as often as we could. We found solace walking the grounds of nearby Tanglewood and had our unwinding sessions in favorite restaurants. We also developed special friendships with many people who were so kind to us.

Throughout this time, with frequent trips to the

Berkshires, when the situation was hectic and exhausting both mentally and physically, I functioned quite well. It was truly amazing, because as soon as we were either settled in a motel for the evening or back home, my G.I. tract would go wild and keep me up all night. But I was given the time to do what was needed of me, for which I am most grateful.

As all these events were taking place in the Berkshire area, Russ's mother was beginning to decline in health. She lived alone in Cummington, about twenty- five miles away from Van. We made arrangements for her to move to a winter residence for several years, then we moved her back to Cummington where she did fairly well in the summer enjoying her house. Eventually she had falls and fractures and finally needed care in a nursing home. This facility was about fifty miles from Lenox and we tended to her needs as well as we could. Following a massive stroke in 1988, she died in 1989 at the age of ninety.

Russ and I have maintained her house, which has become a refuge for us when we are able to get away for a few days during the summer. This is one of the loveliest spots in the Berkshires and one of my "healing places."

Every three months I returned to Dr. Barton for my checkup. Just before each appointment was due, I felt as if everything was falling apart, but after my exam and a clean bill of health, I always came home revitalized, mentally and physically and ready to take on the world . . .

Many happy events took place during the years following 1986. On Labor Day weekend of 1988, our daughter Sue remarried. She and Bob had a small wedding in a tiny country church in rural Pittsburg, New Hampshire, near their little "getaway" lodge. This was one of my long and worrisome trips on a road where facilities were few and far between. The wedding was lovely and we had no major mishaps other than a bee sting on my hand.

The next happy event was the birth of our first grandson, Cory Paul Landroche, born to Nancy and Jeff in March 1990.

The following April, Jay and Joanne were married. It was nice to be mother of the groom for a change. Planning ahead was difficult for me, as I seemed to have alternating good and bad days. One day I would function fairly well and the next day I might not be able to leave the house.

I tried not to let fear enter into the planning and attending of the pre-nuptial events, including the rehearsal dinner, all held out of town. I tried to juggle in my mind whether I'd actually be able to attend my son's wedding. I couldn't admit this fear to my family, but I was rather tense, which I'm sure didn't help my problems. To ease my mind, we had a hotel room near the reception, even though the wedding was only about forty miles from home. We used it to dress and it was a great place for Jay to pace the floor before the ceremony.

I managed the wedding and reception quite well. Having the hotel room available was a blessing after the festivities were over, but rather than stay the night, Russ and I decided to "run for it" and spend the night in our own bed. How very grateful I was that I was given the blessing of being with my family on this wonderful occasion.

The following year, Jay and Joanne presented us with a new grandson, Brian Joseph, and just before Christmas in

1992, their second son, David Russell Van Billiard, arrived. We were now blessed with five beautiful healthy grandchildren!

A very special event in my life occurred in February 1991. My family and special friends joined together and had a surprise party for me to celebrate my five years as a survivor. I was touched beyond belief and became even more resolved to be around, but not only for another five years. I decided I'd aim for one hundred.

Early in 1993, I mustered up enough courage to suggest a winter vacation. The only comfortable place where I could "get my feet wet" was Key West. I had yearned to return to our first home, where Russ had been stationed with the U.S. Navy and where our first two children, Nancy and Susan, were born.

I hadn't traveled very far with my colostomy and wasn't sure how it would "fly," but in March we made the trip. Although Key West was hardly the quiet, undiscovered town we had known, we soon realized that, even in the midst of "spring break," we loved it as much as ever. We revisited our old homes, other familiar places, and saw a few friends with whom we had kept in touch. It was truly a nostalgic trip and we knew we would continue to return to this tiny paradise, crazy as it was!

We have continued to visit Key West, staying longer each time. Although this island is renowned for its spectacular sunsets, we were more in awe at the sight of the sun rising up out of the ocean in full glory each morning as we watched from our balcony.

Ovarian Cancer
The Disease

Causes

Certain factors are associated with an increased risk of developing ovarian cancer. In some cases, there is a genetic predisposition to the disease. In those with no known genetic factor, there are many hypotheses as to what may cause this disease, although the specific cause or causes are not known.

Evidence from various sources shows that the majority of cases of ovarian cancer occur between the ages of sixty and sixty-nine. Other statistics show that the fifties are the average age, but this does not mean that younger women should be complacent and think they are immune. I was diagnosed at age fifty-six. Over the last twelve years, there have been ten women with ovarian cancer whom I have tried to help in a supportive role and several others whose lives have touched mine indirectly. Their ages ranged from thirty-four to sixty-nine.

Studies indicate that white women seem to be at a slightly higher risk than black women, as are women who have had cancer of the breast or endometrium.

A Canadian study written up in *Prevention Report, U.S. Public Health Service,* October-November 1994, shows that the risk of ovarian cancer rose 20 percent for every ten grams of saturated fat consumed daily. Unsaturated fat apparently did not add to the risk. Adding ten grams of vegetable fiber lowered the risk of ovarian cancer by 37 percent.

An article in the *Journal of Clinical Oncology*, vol.13, no.3, March 1995, states that reproductive and environmental factors may contribute to the development of ovarian cancer. Investigation shows that it would appear that the greater number of ovulatory cycles a woman has, the more her risk increases. Also, women who have not borne children or have had fewer children are at a greater risk, while those women who breast feed, thus prolonging the return of ovulation, and those who use oral contraceptives appear to have a decreased risk for developing ovarian cancer. Fertility drugs such as Clomid and Perganol may also increase the risk.

More recent studies by Dr. Andrew Berchuck, of the Duke University Medical Center, explain that a high number of ovulations increases the chances that p53, a tumor suppressor gene, can be mutated. The majority of ovarian cancers have the p53 mutation, which occurs due to ovulation.

Another possible cause of ovarian cancer is the use of talcum powder on perineal pads or in the perineal area, although this theory is now being discounted.

Studies show that ovarian cancer affects women of all prosperous industrialized countries, excluding Japan. These women have a greater exposure to carcinogenic material. Dr. M. Steven Piver, chief of the department of gynecological oncology at the Roswell Park Cancer Institute, explains that the use of asbestos-containing talc can be a possible cause of ovarian cancer, as the talc particles can travel upward through the vagina and uterus to the ovaries in the same manner as sperm travels. But again, this theory has few proponents.

Even though Japan is an industrialized nation, the incidence of cancer there is low. According to Dr. Piver, the diet in Japan is low in fat, yet when Japanese women move to the United States and change to a typically Western high-fat diet, the incidence becomes the same as for American women.

While there has not been any data implicating some of the risk factors we relate to the development of cancer, such as smoking and alcohol consumption, diet may well be an important factor.

An article by Carol Potera in *Longevity* states that researchers at the University of California, San Diego, found that women from ages forty-five to fifty-four who live in the northern part of the United States had a higher incidence of ovarian cancer than those women living in the southern states. It is "hypothesized that they have a shortage of vitamin D" resulting from too little exposure to the sun. Including food rich in vitamin D and drinking fortified milk can help meet the recommended daily allowance of 400 I.U.'s.

Also in this article was a report of a preliminary study by researchers at Boston's Brigham and Women's Hospital. This study found that women who took tricyclic antidepressants such as Valium, Halcion, and Elavil "doubled their risk for ovarian cancer, and if they used the drugs before age fifty, they carried up to 3.5 times the normal risk." It was concluded that further studies are needed.

Researchers from Brigham and Women's Hospital are currently attempting to establish a link between the use of acetaminophen and ovarian cancer. This medication, used in several over-the-counter painkillers, might lower the risk of developing this disease.

While none of these causative theories has been confirmed, the genetic theory has been proved factual.

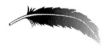

The Genetic Factor

In addition to the p53 suppressor gene mutation due to a high number of ovulations, there are other important genetic factors. According to Henry T. Lynch and others, of Creighton University's Hereditary Cancer Institute, "About one in seventy women in the United States will manifest ovarian carcinoma during their lifetimes." Of all the gynecological malignancies, ovarian cancer has the highest mortality rate.

Dr. Lynch believes that familial ovarian cancer is a "crude way of estimating cancer risk to relatives of cancer affecteds. It has been variably defined as occurring in a single first-degree relative plus one or more second-degree relatives." A proband is the initial member of a family to be studied for an inherited trait or disease.This familial concept does not emphasize the importance of some of the clinical features of hereditary ovarian cancer's natural history, such as "age of onset, cancers of other anatomic sites, or multiple cancer patterns."

Dr. Lynch also explains the familial risk may be attributed to some of the "common familiar environment exposures and to genetic factors" that may not have a significant effect on the risk. However, studies of families demonstrating hereditary cancer show that some genes have a major effect on the ovarian cancer risk. It is a fact that "having a single first-degree relative with ovarian cancer increases the lifetime risk for this disease."

Two important hereditary disorders associated with ovarian cancer, hereditary breast/ovarian (HBOC) and hereditary nonpolyposis colorectal cancer (HNPCC or the Lynch Syndrome), are known to be due to primary genetic factors.

According to Drs. Susan E. Mackey and William T. Creasman of the Department of Obstetrics and Gynecology at the Medical College of South Carolina, as the risk factors were studied and developed from cancer-prone families, an autosomal dominant pattern of inheritance was found.

These patterns are divided into three subsets:

(1) site-specific familial cancer associated only with epithelial ovarian cancer

(2) breast/ovarian familial cancer syndrome, which includes both breast and epithelial ovarian cancer

(3) Lynch II Syndrome associated with familial clustering of breast, ovarian, endometrial, gastrointestinal, and genitourinary cancers

Mackey and Creasman explain, "In all three types, males are felt to be capable of carrying the affected gene with the degree of risk to an individual patient dependent on the frequency of the occurrence of cancer in first and second-degree relatives."

There are in-depth studies available that explain the complexities of the genetic epidemiology of ovarian cancer. I am not including this precise scientific data, since it does not seem appropriate in a book of this type.

In the manuscript made available to me by Dr. Lynch,

there are some recommendations regarding genetic counseling. Ideally, this counseling should be performed by the family physician, provided he or she understands the principles of genetics and the natural history of hereditary cancer. This counseling should be reinforced by other members of the team including the gynecologist and the oncologist, and, when necessary, a referral to a cancer geneticist. When possible, this counseling should be provided to all high-risk members of the family, as well as the patient, and should be adapted to the patient's level of understanding. Such counseling has been provided to ovarian cancer-prone families over the past several decades by Dr. Lynch and associates at Creighton University.

Because the surveillance presently available is not good, Dr. Lynch recommends that prophylactic oophorectomy (removal of the ovaries) be a strong consideration in "patients who are carriers of the BRCA 1 gene in the HBOC syndrome."

Another source of information regarding hereditary ovarian cancer is the Familial Ovarian Cancer Registry, which was established in 1981 by M. Steven Piver, M.D., chief of the Department of Gynecologic Oncology at Roswell Park Cancer Institute. After the death from ovarian cancer of comedienne Gilda Radner, the institute was renamed to honor her memory. The registry now has about one thousand women listed who have been diagnosed with ovarian cancer in more than four hundred families with two or more members with ovarian cancer.

This registry can be most helpful in aiding a family's

search for a familial link to the disease, as the identifications of those cancer patients include the women's married and maiden names, as well as other relevant data.

Data from the Roswell Park Institute also discusses prophylactic oophorectomy and recommends that women with a family history of ovarian cancer undergo this surgery by age thirty-five if they have completed their family. This is done by video laparoscopy and allows for thorough examination of the pelvic and abdominal areas. Also, both ovaries should be carefully evaluated pathologically to be certain that no very small ovarian cancer is present.

In recommending this prophylactic, or preventive, procedure, there has been concern that papillary carcinoma of the peritoneum (lining of the abdominal cavity) could develop ("with the histologic appearance of ovarian cancer"). This has occurred in a small number of women who have undergone this prophylactic oophorectomy due to a familial history of ovarian cancer. While the risk is small, it is certainly a consideration.

In some ethnic groups such as Ashkenazi Jews from eastern and central europe, a greater proportion of ovarian cancers is inherited (around 3 in 10). There are several genetic factors that increase the risk of ovarian cancer. Several mutations in BRCA1 and BRCA2 have been observed to occur with a higher frequency among these individuals of Ashkenazi Jewish descent.

For women at risk, physical surveillance should consist of pelvic and abdominal examination, CA 125, and transvaginal ultrasound every six months.

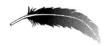

Screening

Unfortunately, the surveillance methods for discovering early ovarian cancer and the associated risk factors are not good. Most cases diagnosed early and still localized are identified by chance. Earlier methods used in an attempt to screen for precancerous and early-stage malignant disease were unsuccessful and are no longer used.

Methods being explored today as potential screening tools include the use of tumor markers, specifically the CA 125, transvaginal ultrasonography, and color Doppler imaging.

Major obstacles in early detection are that the disease is asymptomatic in the early stages and the lack of information or understanding about the natural history of ovarian cancer. Mackey and Creasman explain that "it is generally assumed to progress in an orderly fashion from stage I to stage IV, although the length of time spent in each stage is unknown." There is also controversy as to whether ovarian cysts are potentially malignant. There appears to be no documentation regarding the presence of a premalignant stage for ovarian cancer.

Screening tests should meet certain criteria, such as being fairly simple, safe, and reasonably painless procedures. These tests should also be inexpensive and valid. As explained by Mackey and Creasman, the validity of a screening test is measured by its sensitivity, specificity, and predictive values. The sensitivity indicates the probability that the test will be positive when the disease is present; specificity represents the probability that the test will be negative when there is no disease present. Importantly, say Mackey and Creasman, the positive predictive value "represents the number of diagnostic procedures performed on patients without the disease for every procedure performed on patients with the disease."

Transabdominal ultrasonography had many disadvantages, including a high false positive rate. This means that about fifty abdominal surgical procedures (laparotomies) would be necessary to discover one case of primary ovarian cancer. In an attempt to improve on the transabdominal type, the transvaginal ultrasonography was investigated for screening. In this method, a probe placed in the vagina scans the ovaries for tumors, but is not accurate in differentiating benign from malignant tumors.

Transvaginal color Doppling detects abnormal blood flow to the ovaries. Since ovarian cancers develop new blood vessels, this test may identify the new blood vessel formation.

A tumor marker, CA 125, is a blood test, or assay, that measures the presence of ovarian tumor antigen present in most patients with ovarian cancer. While it is most useful in monitoring the treatment of ovarian cancer and detecting a recurrence, this test cannot be used by itself for routine screening.

Several conditions could cause the CA 125 to be elevated, resulting in a false positive. Because of many variables, an early tumor could be missed; and some women could be given the false reassurance that they have no malignancy based on this test alone.

Studies seem to show that the most useful method of screening is transvaginal sonography, possibly with color Doppler imaging. The procedure is fairly simple and seems to be highly specific and sensitive. Routine screening, however, is not feasible at this time. Screening for those women at risk who have a family history is appropriate and recommended, but this group represents less than 1 percent of all ovarian cancer patients, according to one study. (Other researchers believe that this group is between 5 and 10 percent.)

Since prevalence of ovarian cancer is fairly low, and the poor success of routine screening methods, some experts in this field suggest that it would be more efficient to emphasize prevention through the use of oral contraceptives, tubal ligations, and removal of the ovaries if the need for a hysterectomy arises. I would think that reducing fat intake might be worthwhile, as well.

Symptoms

The most common type of ovarian cancer, epithelial carcinoma, occurs in the epithelium, or lining, of the ovary. This is the type I will describe. It represents about 18 percent of all gynecological malignancies and is quite possibly the most frequent cause of cancer death in women. Presumably, half of all cases occur in women over the age of sixty-five, although the peak incidence is considered to be in women between the ages of fifty-five and fifty-nine.

I hesitate to use these statistics, and have not been comfortable using any statistics throughout this book, because in every aspect of this disease that I have researched, I have found a varied or wide statistical range. There is much we need to learn about ovarian cancer before we can begin to get the best of it.

Of course, early diagnosis offers the best hope for survival but, as has been discussed, this is extremely difficult. Unfortunately, there are few or no symptoms until the cancer has progressed and enlarged enough to produce symptoms, thus the name "silent killer." Some of these symptoms include abdominal bloating or swelling, vague discomfort in the lower abdomen, feeling full after a light meal, nausea or vomiting, loss of appetite, gas, indigestion, weight loss, diarrhea or constipation, or, less commonly, inappropriate intermittent vaginal bleeding not related to menstrual periods. Often overwhelming fatigue and general malaise are experienced.

Later in the course of the disease, a woman becomes cachexic, or generally emaciated and anemic. At this point, a solid fixed mass can usually be found by pelvic exam. When some of the earlier symptoms do surface, because they are of a nature that could relate to many other medical problems, both minor and serious, it is easy to see that these symptoms could often be mistaken for other ailments. This accounts for the difficulty and frequent delay in diagnosing ovarian cancer.

Usually the cancer is not discovered until it has spread to other organs, including the bowel and liver. As this tumor grows, pressure on the bladder and bowel increases, causing frequent urination and constipation. These symptoms could easily be attributed to a gastrointestinal virus, gastroenteritis, irritable colon, even a urinary tract infection. Other areas of the body where the tumor can spread before diagnosis include the stomach and diaphragm, which can cause shortness of breath. This results in fluid buildup in the abdomen, causing noticeable swelling known as ascites.

Metastasis occurs when the cancer cells enter the bloodstream and the lymphatic system and spread to other parts of the body. By then, this condition can be detected by examining fluid removed from the abdomen and pleural (chest) area, as well as by X-rays and/or scans showing distant metastasis to lung and bone.

In the case of Gilda Radner, her complaints had included debilitating fatigue and general malaise, both attributed by her physician to depression, since no other cause had been found during physical examination.

Ten months later, after she had developed many more symptoms, which had been attributed to various ailments including a viral infection such as Epstein-Barr (which causes overwhelming fatigue), she was again given to believe that her illness was stress-related depression and anxiety. Not until her cancer had spread to her liver and bowel was Gilda's malignancy discovered.

At this time she was suffering from a low-grade fever, pelvic cramping, swelling of the abdomen, and gas, as well as aches and pains in her legs and upper thighs. Interestingly enough, her blood tests, barium enemas, and pelvic ultrasound exams were not consistent with any serious disease.

As I mentioned previously, my first symptom was vaginal spotting in April 1985, which was apparently disregarded, as an endometrial biopsy and pelvic exam done at this time reported negative findings. The pelvic mass, attributed to a large uterine "fibroid," was found in October 1985 during a routine exam. The intestinal obstruction, which was due to the spread of the cancer to my small bowel, was attributed to either the "fibroid" or—who knows? Perhaps the groin discomfort was a sign.

It was not until about two weeks prior to my scheduled "hysterectomy," mid-January 1986, that I began to notice bowel changes, pressure and discomfort after my evening meal, and, finally, abdominal swelling. All in all, I really had no reason to believe that I had ovarian cancer until I developed abdominal swelling. If the ultrasounds had not been negative, I would have run for help, but I trusted those caring for me at the time.

Among the women with ovarian cancer with whom I developed some type of supportive relationship, they all had experienced a varied set of symptoms. None of these symptoms caused any one of them to suspect that she had cancer, according to the stories the women related.

One woman was stricken with severe abdominal pain and rushed to a hospital, where her surgery was performed as an emergency. Later attempts to prolong her life were carried out in a large medical center, but were unsuccessful.

Another victim of the disease first experienced shortness of breath. This sent her to her local physician, who proceeded with diagnostic measures that indicated ovarian cancer. A third woman noticed as the first sign that her abdomen was becoming larger, where previously she had a flat "stomach." She apparently mentioned this with no great concern when she presented herself for a routine physical. Another woman, in her early forties, told me she had no symptoms and had passed her annual gynecological examination with flying colors only weeks before symptoms developed. She then returned to her physician, a diagnosis of ovarian cancer was made, and surgery was performed.

Noting that a great number of women who develop ovarian cancer are in their sixties, I emphasize the importance of continuing regular gynecological examinations. In postmenopausal women, ovaries are small and not usually felt during a pelvic examination. Any ovarian enlargement in these postmenopausal women should trigger the alarm that a malignancy may well be present.

The description of symptoms is unsettling and extremely frightening. In a message of hope to women, including such a depressing chapter may seem counterproductive; yet this may be the most important message I can give. Because most women experience some of these symptoms at some time in their lives, they should by all means have them checked out, no matter how trivial they seem. It is far better to be considered a hypochondriac than to be a victim of ovarian cancer!

Treatment, Staging, and Prognosis

According to The National Cancer Institute's publication *PDQ*, the treatment of ovarian cancer is evolving rapidly, so patients with this disease should be considered as candidates for clinical trials. When a woman is suspected of having ovarian cancer and surgery is to be scheduled, she must make the most important and informed decision of her life. She must decide who will perform her surgery.

Since there is considerable evidence that the amount of disease left in the body at the completion of the primary surgical procedure is related to the patient's survival, it is crucial to select the best qualified surgeon, one who has a "proven track record" in this specialty. There are oncological gynecologists in many of the larger medical centers who are highly skilled and experienced in debulking (removing all or as much as possible of the cancer). In an abstract from the *Archives of Gynecology and Obstetrics*, it was concluded that "only patients with optimally resected Stage III or IV ovarian cancer have a realistic chance of long-term survival."

To women who suspect that they may have ovarian cancer or who have been positively diagnosed, I stress the importance of seeking out the very best care, regardless of how far they must travel. Their survival may depend on it.

At the 1996 annual meeting of the American Society for Clinical Oncology, a National Cancer Institute study found that 90 percent of women having surgery for early-stage ovarian cancer were not thoroughly checked to see if the disease had spread. This omission can mean the difference between life and death. The major reason given by the physicians who documented this study was ignorance among surgeons regarding how this deadly cancer metastasizes throughout the body.

The stage of ovarian cancer refers to how far the disease has advanced. Staging is determined during the primary surgery, and treatment is planned accordingly. There are four stages of ovarian cancer: I, II, III, and IV, each further classified as A, B, or C. A simplified description of these stages is as follows:

The disease is limited to one or both ovaries in Stage I. In Stage II the cancer has spread beyond the ovaries but has not gone outside the pelvic area. In Stage III the cancer has spread to other parts of the abdomen or to lymph nodes. Stage IV has spread more extensively and usually involves the inside of the liver.

The prognosis worsens as the stage increases, but I am not including any statistics on survival rates. I had decided to be one of the survivors, and I think that is the more positive approach! My cancer was Stage III C, and I beat the odds!

In all stages of the disease, surgery is the first treatment. In selected patients with Stage I, where only one ovary is cancerous and the woman wishes to have children at a later time, sometimes the unaffected ovary, fallopian tube, and uterus are left intact, although pelvic tissues are biopsied.

In all other stages of the disease, the surgical procedure involves the removal of the pelvic organs—both ovaries, fallopian tubes, uterus, and the omentum. (The omentum is the part of the tissue that stretches from the stomach to nearly all organs in the abdomen.) Lymph nodes and other tissues are biopsied. In addition, optimal debulking must be done at this time.

Surgery is followed by chemotherapy, either intravenously, by pill, or directly into the abdominal cavity. In some cases, radiation therapy may be prescribed. The treatment depends on the stage of the disease.

The ordeal of chemotherapy, with all its horror stories, is not nearly as dreadful today. There are newer drugs available to lessen the nausea and vomiting that were so devastating to me. Two such medications are Zofran (ondansetron) and Ativan.

Two other therapeutic drugs are Neupogen and Epogen. Neupogen, G-CSF (granulocyte colony-stimulating factor) is given to decrease the incidence of infection during the course of chemotherapy. Anticancer drugs greatly lower the number of white blood cells, increasing the risks of infection. Since chemotherapy cannot be given when the white blood cell count has dropped below a certain level, there were many times when treatments had to be postponed. Neupogen increases the white blood cell count and maintains the proper blood level during this time when a patient's immune system is compromised. Epogen is a drug that stimulates the production of red blood cells and is used to treat or prevent anemia in patients who are undergoing chemotherapy. This drug reduces the need for transfusions in many of these cases.

As to the chemotherapy itself, it is given according to a prescribed protocol depending on the stage of the disease and other factors. The anticancer drugs used primarily in various combinations for ovarian cancer are cyclophosphamide (Cytoxan), cisplatin (Platinol), carboplatin (Paraplatin), and doxorubicin (Adriamycin). Another drug is Hexalen. Protocols, or regimens, which include combinations of these drugs, are considered to be first-line drugs.

Taxol (paclitaxel), an extract of the bark of the Pacific yew and later synthesized, was approved in 1992 for advanced cases of ovarian cancer that had not responded to other therapies or had progressed after treatment. It is now being used as a first-line drug, particularly in combination with cisplatin.

Early in 1996, topotecan (Hycamtin) became available. Topotecan is a valuable new anticancer agent now being used for the treatment of patients with advanced ovarian cancer after failure of the initial or subsequent chemotherapy with cisplatin, carboplatin, or paclitaxel (Taxol).

Hycamtin is a semisynthetic derivative of campothecin, which comes from what is called the Chinese tree of joy. This tree is not lovely to look at—it resembles a scrub pine—but it is now grown in the United States and readily available.

Based on a pilot study conducted at Memorial Sloan-Kettering in New York, a national research organization known as the Gynecolocial Oncology Group is opening a prospective trial of dose-intense chemotherapy for newly diagnosed ovarian cancer patients. This protocol uses high doses of Taxol and carboplatin administered at two-week intervals supported by autologous stem-cell transplantation.

T-stem cells are derived from bone marrow. They go through a process of division and maturation to become specialized types of lymphocytes necessary to fight cancer cells. These stem cells are harvested (removed) from the patient prior to chemotherapy so that they are not killed by the extremely high doses of chemo-therapeutic drugs. Later, they are transplanted back to the patient. Such removal and subsequent return of a person's cells or blood is called an autologous donation.

Another new drug that could be a godsend to patients receiving cisplatin is amifostine (Ethyol). This is a chemo-protective drug used to overcome the toxic effects of cisplatin, one of which is peripheral neuropathy—a debilitating loss of function in the extremities.

We cannot ignore the fact that spontaneous remissions and miracles occur.

> "Miracles are not contrary to nature, but only contrary to what we know about nature."
> —St. Augustine of Hippo (354 - 430 A.D.)

While I had a "second-look" laparotomy at the completion of my chemotherapy, Dr. Barton says that this is rarely done now. It is indicated only when a patient is on an experimental chemotherapy protocol and there is a rise in the CA 125. If, however, one of Dr. Barton's patients later has the need for unrelated abdominal surgery, he is present during the surgery to do a "second look" and cell washings in the abdominal cavity to be sure there are no cancer cells lurking inside.

Though not a positive thought, cancer does recur in a number of patients even when the second-look surgery shows no disease and a negative CA 125 exists. Should recurrent disease develop, there are several options for treatment now under clinical evaluation, particularly for disease that has been resistant to the types of chemotherapy previously used.

As I update this book in 2005, having survived nearly twenty years without a recurrence, I am constantly reminded in my research that relapsing disease is a major concern in the treatment of ovarian cancer. It is disheartening that first line treatment has not changed dramatically. Second line treatment includes many protocols, often using multiple drugs.

Ovarian cancer continues to be the leading cause of death attributed to gynecologic malignancies. While the number of new cases seems to remain stable, early detection and treatment is increasing the five-year survival rate among women diagnosed with this disease. A great number of patients respond to first line therapy only to relapse within the next two years. But the encouraging news, according to Dr. Theodore C. Barton, is that over fifty percent have responded with significant secondary responses and /or remissions. The efficacy of the treatment may thus be approaching that observed for certain chronic diseases such as heart failure, colorectal cancer, some of the hematologic malignancies, and diabetes. This treatment may allow a woman to enjoy her life with reasonably good quality while adding to her longevity.

What has emerged is an ever - expanding area of clinical trials developed and improving daily to allow those women with ovarian cancer who have recurrent disease to be more hopeful. There are trials and phases for which a woman who has had a recurrence may qualify. If this treatment brings her into a complete remission for a period of time where she can function at a nearly normal or above level of activity and good health and then has another recurrence, there are still new trials in the pipeline.

Exciting and encouraging information regarding clinical trials has been given to me by Richard T. Penson, MRCP MD, Clinical Director, Medical Gynecologic Oncology, Massachusetts General Hospital. Clinical trials are studies of new drugs to clarify side effects and see what dose is best (Phase I), see how effective the new drug is (Phase II) and compare a promising drug with standard treatment (Phase III).

At the present time, three strategies are being investigated in an attempt to improve survival outcomes for women with advanced ovarian cancer. Intraperitoneal therapy has been investigated for decades, and there are now three randomized controlled trials (Phase III), which demonstrate at least delayed recurrence and perhaps improved survival, with chemotherapy given directly into the abdominal cavity. However, it is not clear that the improvement in overall survival outweighs the increased toxicity, which has prevented intraperitoneal administration becoming a routine part of clinical care. Secondly, many of the agents that are active in recurrent disease are being investigated. In the five-arm national study, GOG 182, topotecan, gemcitabine and Doxil are being combined with carboplatin and paclitaxel. Lastly, the biologics: Interferon Gamma, oral Epidermal Growth Factor

Inhibitors (such as Iressa and Tarceva), monoclonal antibodies and radioimmunotherapeutics are all being investigated. For example, Pemtumomab (Theragyn) is a combination of an antibody against a mucin (Sugar-protein cellular defense) on the surface of ovarian cancer cells and has attached to it, a molecule of the radioactive metal, Yttrium. The hope is that a single intraperitoneal treatment after the completion of first line chemotherapy will eradicate microscopic residual cells to which the antibody binds. Other immunotherapies include GM-CSF, IL-2 and IFNg. Progress with vaccines continues to be slow. Gene therapy is even more of a challenge, but antiangiogenic therapies, designed to target the developing blood supply of the cancer got a tremendous boost at the 2003 American Society of Clinical Oncology (ASCO) meeting, with the first evidence that the addition of a new antibody, bevacizumab (Avastin), targeted at Vascular Endothelial Growth Factor (VEGF) Receptors, to chemotherapy increased survival in patients with cancer. VEGF probably plays an important role in ovarian cancer behavior and this is definitely an area to watch. Antiangiogenic drugs being investigated for ovarian cancer include Squalamine, CAI and NM-3.

Two therapies that recently entered large, randomized Phase III trials are OvaRex and Telcyta (previously called TLK286). OvaRex is an antibody that binds to the tumor marker CA-125 to try and provoke the patient's immune system to fight the cancer, and Telcyta is a novel prodrug that is activated by the patient's metabolism to kill cancer. In Phase II clinical trials, the Taxol-like drugs CT2103 and Tularik, Irofulven (MGI-114), Velcade (PS-341), Tirapazamine, Phenoxodiol, and Yondelis (ET-743) all are exciting new compounds and there are in excess of 800 new agents in Phase I clinical trials in the United States.

Cancer is frightening. Many ovarian cancer patients become addicted to their CA-125, "if it's OK, I'm OK." In the fight against cancer, you are more important than your disease. Don't let it define you. Living with cancer is all about making the most important things in your life count. The theme of the 2003 ASCO Annual Meeting was Commitment. Care. Compassion: Honoring People with Cancer. There are wonderful advocacy programs. One in Boston is O.C.E.A.N. (The Ovarian Cancer Education and Awareness Network). There are also many national organizations that can be contacted through the World Wide Web, such as *Conversations*, and the National Ovarian Cancer Coalition (NOCC).

According to Dr. Penson, who addresses the question, 'how you can contribute to being a survivor?' "Be proactive in making goals of your dreams and facing your responsibilities. Make sure you are well supported. Find the best doctors and the best care. Resource yourself with clear information. Knowing more will increase your confidence. There are many survivors who have been through exactly what you are experiencing. Although we don't know the answers to many of the questions that face us with cancer, together thousands of women can find a voice and keep hope alive. A feather in all of their hats."

As this book is meant to give hope to those women with ovarian cancer and their loved ones, I have done much soul searching as how to bring readers up to a realistic approach to current treatment and prognosis without diminishing the very guts of my book—*the fight to survive.*

Outlook

The Effects of Managed Care

Will we ever find a way to conquer ovarian cancer? If so, will it be by discovering the cause? by prevention? by a new effective screening method? a miracle cure? No one knows, but I am hopeful.

Overshadowing my hope, though, is skepticism due to a fast-developing trend affecting the delivery of health care known as managed health care. This health insurance system is forcing the medical profession, allied health professionals, and hospitals to compromise their standards of care and ethics.

Not only is the quality and quantity of patient care being directed by insurance companies, instead of by physicians, but also research de facto is being neglected. For instance, according to a special investigation by *Time* magazine, a large California health plan, Health Net, threw out a proposal to allocate funds for the study of ovarian cancer. The grounds were that such an investment might put the company at risk, under the Americans with Disabilities Act, of being accused of discriminating against people with other diseases. As Health Net's vice president for legal services said, "If we put money into ovarian cancer research and word gets out, then it isn't going to be long before AIDS groups or prostate cancer groups start having a field day."

Ovarian cancer is such an insidious disease that it is called "the silent killer." It is difficult enough to diagnose and treat by specialists in this field. With "managed care" and its proposals, women may not have access to those with the expertise to save their lives for two reasons.

First, in an article in the *New England Journal of Medicine,* a new plan is being considered that ties doctors' incomes to curtailing service. The new "risk-sharing" arrangements would allow participating physicians to profit from not referring patients.

Second, in a recent *Bulletin of the American College of Surgeons,* an article discussing the ethical dilemmas involved in managed care shows that nothing can hide the fact that 35 percent of premiums spent will be expended on "matters other than the patient." This figure represents expenses for "administration, income tax, and profit." This can apparently be achieved only by denial of services or, as Dr. Fischer calls it, "rationing (the R word), or by substituting generalists for specialists."

Dr. Fischer writes that in selling managed care to the public, several assumptions have been postulated. Two that I recognize as having a negative impact on the diagnosis and treatment of ovarian cancer are:

> "Physician extenders can recognize illness as easily and as completely as specialists."

> "Generalists are as competent in recognizing and treating serious illness as specialists."

Many patients have not been referred to specialists

until it is too late because of the added cost to the HMO. Too bad that "the bottom line" is more important than "the cutting edge."

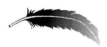

Closure

On Being Cured

As the saying goes—you never know when you'll hit the long ball out of the park . . .

On September 27, 1995, I had an appointment with Dr. Barton. After examining me, he deferred my CA 125 and told me that I was "CURED."

Cured is a powerful word! Hearing it from Dr. Barton was the culmination of the battle I had been fighting and the affirmation that I had won. However, this news did not mean that I would let down my defenses, because I will always be vigilant and commune daily with Thaddeus and his horde of TLCs. I continue my quarterly exams with Dr. Barton and have an annual CA 125 and mammogram.

I am always endeavoring to redefine the priorities in my life and become more adaptable in some of the situations where I easily lose patience. Every so often I allow foolish, inconsequential things to overwhelm me, when plans go wrong and I feel that I no longer control my life. Then I attempt to break loose from such rigidity. I forget too easily how I had, for a while, let trivial matters slide by me, focusing only on the preciousness of life, savoring every moment and grateful to get out of bed each morning.

When we are faced with a life-threatening illness and the outlook is uncertain, no matter how positive an attitude we may have, we tend to develop an urgent awareness of the sanctity of life. We direct our energies toward grasping each moment and experiencing every simple day-to-day event eagerly, wishing we could hang on to it forever. Nothing else seems important other than being alive. Then, when at last we find ourselves "out of the woods," how easy it is to slip back into the old rigid scheme of things; we tend to revert to our old attitudes and schedules and let the roses go to seed, unnoticed, the lovely fragrance gone by. While this is not good, it is part of the human condition.

We can't go through the rest of our lives with a constant smile on our faces ignoring the realities of everyday living. But when we are SURVIVORS, it shouldn't be too difficult—nor cause us to be the objects of criticism—to reclaim that Cheshire-cat grin that says, "I did it!"

After a few months of basking in the joy of my triumph, I went for my regular checkup with Dr. Barton. I learned that there was a chink in my armor; fortunately, nothing serious, but what had previously been a weakened area in my large abdominal muscle due to five surgical incisions was now a real cleft known as a ventral hernia. When Dr. Barton told me that this hernia should be repaired, I told him that I would never return to an operating room unless I were bound, gagged, and dragged. After such badinage, I realized that I really had no choice. I needed to have the job done, but I deferred scheduling the procedure until after our trip to Key West.

This vacation was very special, as we took our daughter Nancy to spend the first five days with us. It was a dream fulfilled. Nancy, our firstborn, was a true "Key West Conch," as the natives are called, born in the U.S. Naval

Hospital there. She had never returned to her birthplace. Our visit was truly a spiritual experience and as such I did not want to cast any pall over this joyful occasion by mentioning or even thinking about impending surgery. Surprisingly enough, my inner strength, girded by prayer and Thaddeus, enabled me to suppress all of my concerns and not waste a single happy moment.

In May, I entered the New England Baptist Hospital and enthusiastically submitted to have my worn-out tummy muscles replaced with some type of plastic, technically known as Prolene. I was now anticipating with pleasure having my sagging belly remodeled.

Upon waking from anesthesia, Dr. Barton told me that the surgery went well, then added jokingly, "I have good news and bad news." The good news was that the repair was so extensive that a "tummy tuck" was necessary. The bad news: I was now "like Eve"—I no longer had a belly button. I thought to myself, "So what! That's the least of my worries!"

When Russ and Nancy visited me at the hospital, Nancy said, "Never mind, Mom, if you ever need a belly button, you can always draw one on with a Magic Marker."

That summer, for the first time in my life, I wore a bikini in the privacy of our pool. Lest anyone catch me, there was a small circle with a smile drawn in the middle with a small, felt-tipped pen, right where it belonged.

I am often questioned about my daily living habits, mostly by other cancer patients or those interested in my survival techniques. I have never tried any macrobiotic or fad diets, nor have I consumed any of the various foods or concoctions credited with suppressing or slowing down the cancer process. There are foods I can no longer tolerate, because of extensive bowel surgery. I also developed a severely irritable colon. There are times when cravings get the better of me and I indulge in the forbidden foods. Usually it's worth the resulting discomfort. Most of the time, I eat a healthy diet that includes lots of broiled fish, chicken, salad, fruit, and good bread and pasta. I can't live without pizza and occasionally crash and burn on Mexican, Asian, and other ethnic foods.

I enjoy a cocktail or two before dinner or a glass of red wine. I learned that this is conducive to maintaining a high and healthy HDL component of my cholesterol. This pleases me since I am a cheese lover. Also, by using fat-free ingredients that aren't discernible in cooking, I can indulge in good cheese without guilt.

I gave up smoking about twenty-three years ago, for which I am extremely grateful. I doubt I could have survived had I been a smoker. I learned that smoking and living are not compatible, and I chose life!

Multivitamins and minerals have continued to be a daily supplement to the most adequate diet I enjoy, and I probably don't need them. I do, however, require a thyroid supplement. Since my terminal ileum, the part of the small intestine that absorbs vitamin B12, was removed during my debulking surgery, I require a monthly injection of that vitamin.

Monthly allergy injections are also part of my life. In my younger years, I was allergic to dust and molds and have been treated for over twenty years by Dr. John O'Loughlin of the Lahey Clinic. Not only is he an outstanding allergist and immunologist, but has also shown a special talent in reassuring and offering suggestions to me for other problems I experienced over the years. While it is possible that I may no longer require the allergy injections, I do continue them. Dr. O'Loughlin told me that while there was no proof, there is evidence that the allergy injections could be a factor in maintaining a strong immune system.

Contrary to the advice of dermatologists, I continue to be a lover of the sun. While I am cautious, I do enjoy keeping a healthy-looking tan in the summer and on winter vacations. I can't give up everything that's bad for me. Life is a risk and, as Bette Midler's character said in *The Rose,* "It's the soul afraid of dying that never learns to live." So much for wrinkles!

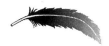

The Next Seven Years

1998-2005

Seven years later, there are many more wrinkles and other visible signs of my victory over ovarian cancer. The invisible signs are the ones that present the greatest obstacles. I try to resolve guilt feelings that push their way in, as I must give up so many significant events. I miss attending my beloved church and participating in its life. I have come to accept that travel to exotic places and certain social activities are out of reach, but this type of life is no longer as important to me as it once was.

In an April 2002 Teleconference entitled, "Management of Ovarian Cancer Treatment Side effects," Michael V. Seiden, MD PhD, of Massachusetts General Hospital in Boston stated that while cure seems to be still elusive, key side effects from ovarian cancer treatment can be dealt with. These side effects include bowel dysfunction, fatigue, pain, neuropathy and stress. In a summary published in *Conversations*, Dr. Seiden explains that," Ovarian cancer is a long - haul disease. With any luck, we're going to be coping with it for a long time and it's a stressful companion."

After living for nearly twenty years with every one of these stressful companions and others as well, I can't say I enjoy their company. But I am very blessed to be alive even with the many encumberances that go along with survivorship. They are ever-present reminders of the disease that is *no longer silent.*

I recall a quote, "From those to whom much has been given, much is expected." Although I'm not sure of the author, I find myself living by this message every day. After the many blessings that I have received, I truly believe that I have been given a mission in my life. To offer help and hope to women afflicted with ovarian cancer seems to be that mission.

Since *Feather* was published, I have met and become personally involved with many women and their families whose lives have been affected by ovarian cancer. Many of these women have actually made the trip to Boston for second opinions and treatment. Some have done well. A few of them, some of whom became dear friends, are now new Angels in Heaven. My grief is heavy for them, but my hope is great for those who are entering this new era of research and clinical trials. A recurrence is not good, but at least there is now hope for survival.

I can only hope that I will be able to continue to be available to those who may need my help. With God's blessings, I pray that I will meet the expectations that have been laid upon me.

LXXIX

Let me not pray to be sheltered from
dangers but to be fearless in facing them.

Let me not beg for the stilling of my pain
but for the heart to conquer it.

Let me not look for allies in life's battlefields
but to my own strength.

Let me not crave in anxious fear to be saved
but hope for the patience to win my freedom.

Grant me that I may not be a coward, feeling
your mercy in my success alone; but let me find
the grasp of your hand in my failure.

—Rabindranath Tagore
"Fruit Gathering"

On the more personal side, life has been good to me and my loved ones.

I could not stay away from operating rooms, and unfortunately have endured three more surgeries, unrelated to my ovarian cancer. I now have two great shoulders thanks to the surgical expertise of Dr. David Mattingly at NEBH who repaired my torn rotater cuffs, and recently I had a spinal fusion performed by Dr. Peter Anas also at NEBH. I am carefully guarding my other joints after being called a "frequent flyer" within the orthopedic community.

For twelve years now we have returned to Key West for four weeks or so in March and feel the emotional attachment to our first home increasing each year. New friendships have been made and old ones nurtured. Somehow, I feel that my physical handicaps are "forgiven" and the laidback Key West lifestyle allows me to relax and promotes healing. It is amazing what a temporary respite from responsibilities can do for a person!

We still don't consider ourselves tourists, but do share their enthusiasm in watching the awesome Key West sunsets. We finally do concede that sunsets can compete with the sunrises in all their splendor, although such magnificant productions, true gifts of God, are not easy to compare. In 2001, we brought our second "conch," daughter Susan, back to visit her birthplace as we had done with Nancy in 1996. Our annual visit to "Paradise" will always be a "key" event.

New family additions include two great-granddaughters, Alison and Ashley Castle, daughters of Sarah and Nathan. Another special "grandson" has entered our lives very unexpectedly. His name is Ijaaz and his name means "miracle." He was born to a young couple, Nizam and Shenaz in Mauritius, an island in the middle of the Indian Ocean. Ijaaz was conceived as a result of this book. My *Feather* flew far away and Nizam found me and asked for help. With the warm and caring collaboration of Dr. Barton and Nancy Bray we acted as a team to turn about the lives of a young family on the other side of the world. This is an incredible story and resulted in the discovery that Shenaz's diagnosis of ovarian cancer was erroneous. So, in March 2000, Ijaaz was born. We keep in touch with this family and receive photos of the important events in the life of Ijaaz.

Russ and I threw caution to the wind and opened our hearts to a kitten, Timothy, who is now five years old and rules our lives. He is some type of tabby from Maine, an anniversary gift from the Landroche family, and has six toes on all four paws, and wing-like markings on his back; thus, we call him our angel kitty. With all four on the floor, he is fast and feisty, but otherwise Timothy is a lovable little guy.

My mother passed away in early 2005 at age ninety-nine. Although her hearing and vision were greatly diminished, her memory was fairly good so we were able to have quite meaningful visits with her. I miss her very much.

Our granddaughter, Lindsay, who wrote "My Grandma" in the beginning of this book, graduated in 2005 from the University of Maine in Orono, Summa Cum Laude, with a degree in elementary education.

Our other grandchildren, Cory, Brian and David, are all doing well and are a source of love and pride.

A big change in my life occurred recently when my two

dear friends, Dr. Ted Barton and Nancy Bray retired. I felt like a lost sheep. This blow was softened somewhat by the fact that over the years we have become very close friends so we see one another quite often.

Dr. Barton left me in the capable hands of a very special physician, a hematologist and oncologist, Dr. Zachary Spigelman whom I have known for several years. He has bailed me out of many medical crises already. Zach is a brilliant, gentle, caring physician and I am grateful to be in his care.

I am truly blessed.

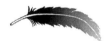

Epilogue

February 10, 2005 was the nineteenth anniversary of my diagnosis and life-saving surgery, with no recurrence of ovarian cancer.

According to Rabbi Harold Kushner, "The Talmud says that there are three things one should do in the course of one's life: have a child, plant a tree, and write a book."

To celebrate my victory, I could plant a mustard seed

> which is indeed the least of all seeds; but when it is grown, it is the greatest among herbs, and becometh a tree, so that the birds of the air come and lodge in the branches thereof.

—Matthew 13:32

LUCINDA MATLOCK

I went to the dances at Chandlerville,
And played snap-out at Winchester.
One time we changed partners,
Driving home in the moonlight of middle June,
And then I found Davis.
We were married and lived together for seventy years,
Enjoying, working, raising the twelve children,
Eight of whom we lost
Ere I had reached the age of sixty.
I spun, I wove, I kept the house, I nursed the sick,
I made the garden, and for holiday
Rambled over the fields where sang the larks,
And by Spoon River gathering many a shell,
And many a flower and medicinal weed—
Shouting to the wooded hills, singing to the green valleys.
At ninety-six I had lived enough, that is all,
And passed to sweet repose.
What is this I hear of sorrow and weariness,
Anger, discontent and drooping hopes?
Degenerate sons and daughters,
Life is too strong for you—
It takes life to love Life.

—Edgar Lee Masters
Spoon River Anthology

This poem hangs in Dr. Barton's examining room and after all these years I know it by heart. I have gained much strength and inspiration from this message, which I interpret in this way:

153

Life is, indeed, too strong for many of us, even though we live in a different era where life should be easier. But with the complexities that accompany this age of high technology, we are pressured to go with the flow. In this frenetic effort to succeed, we often fail to appreciate the preciousness of life until we have nearly lost it. Then, we scramble frantically to make up for lost time, to squeeze out the precious moments we missed along the way.

If only we could slow down and live more passionately while we still have the spark of Life within us.

Bibliography

Benson, Herbert. *Beyond the Relaxation Response*. New York: Times Books, 1984.

———. *The Relaxation Response*. New York: William Morrow, 1975.

Borysenko, Joan. *Fire in the Soul*. New York: Warner Books, 1993.

———. *Minding the Body, Mending the Mind*. New York: Bantam Books, 1988.

Chopra, Deepak. *Ageless Body, Timeless Mind*. New York: Harmony Books, 1993.

Conversations, vol. 10, no. 11. November 2002, p. 8

Cousins, Norman. *Head First, the Biology of Hope*. New York: E.P. Dutton, 1989.

Cramer, Daniel W., Bernard C. Harlow, et al. "Over-the-counter analgesics and risk of ovarian cancer," The *Lancet*, vol. 351, no. 9096, Saturday 10 January 1998, pp. 104–107.

Dossey, Barbara. "Using Imagery to Help Your Patient Heal." *American Journal of Nursing*, vol. 95, no. 6. June 1995, p. 41.

Dossey, Larry. *Meaning and Medicine*. New York: Bantam Books, 1991.

Epstein, Gerald. *Healing Visualizations*. New York: Bantam Books, 1989.

Fain, Jean. "The Silent Killer," *Ladies Home Journal*, March 1990, p. 76.

Faith, Hope and Love—An Inspirational Treasury of Quotations. Philadelphia: Running Press, 1994.

Fischer, Joseph. "Ethical dilemmas in managed care." *Bulletin of the American College of Surgeons,* vol. 80, no. 11, November 1995.

Gouker, Loice. *The Twelve Apostles.* Norwalk: The C.R. Gibson Company, 1960.

Graham, Billy. *Angels.* Dallas: Word Publishing, 1994.

Kübler-Ross, Elisabeth. *On Death and Dying.* New York: The MacMillan Company, 1969.

Kushner, Harold. *When All You've Ever Wanted Isn't Enough.* New York: Pocket Books, 1987.

Larson, Erik. "The Soul of an HMO," *Time.* January 22, 1996, p. 48.

Locke, Steven, and Douglas Colligan. *The Healer Within: The New Medicine of Mind and Body.* New York: Mentor, 1987.

Londer, Randi. "Chemotherapy Goes Circadian," *American Health.* June 1986. pp. 10–11.

Lunt, J., et al.: "Cisplatin Neuropathy with Lhermitte's Sign." *Journal of Neurology, Neurosurgery, and Psychiatry.* 49: 96–99 (March) 1986. Reprinted in *American Journal of Nursing,* (November 1986), p. 1274.

Lynch, Henry T., et al. "Hereditary Ovarian Cancer: Natural History, Surveillance, Management, and Genetic Counseling." *Hematology/Oncology Annals,* vol. 2, no. 2, March/April 1994.

Mackey, Susan E., and William T. Creasman. "Ovarian Cancer Screening," *Journal of Clinical Oncology,* vol.13, no. 3 (March 1995) pp. 783 - 793.

Masters, Edgar Lee. *Spoon River Anthology.* New York: Dover Publications, Inc., 1992.

Matthews-Simonton, Stephanie, O. Carl Simonton, and James L. Creighton. *Getting Well Again.* New York: Bantam Books, 1978.

Naparstek, Belleruth. *Staying Well with Guided Imagery.* New York: Warner Books, 1994.

National Cancer Institute. "PDQ State-of-the-Art Cancer Treatment Summary—Ovarian Epithelial Cancer." 02/95.

————. "PDQ State-of-the-Art Cancer Treatment Summary—Ovarian Epithelial Cancer." 01/98.

Newsletter 1993–94. The Gilda Radner Familial Ovarian Cancer Registry. Roswell Park Cancer Institute, Buffalo, NY.

Potera, Carol, article in *Longevity* (August 1995).

Prevention Report, U.S. Public Health Service. Canadian Report. October–November. 1984, p. 47.

Rothchild, Paul A. and Bill Gazecki. *The Rose.* New York: Atlantic Recording Corp; 1979.

Segal, Marian. "Ovarian Cancer," reprint from *FDA Consumer* Magazine. (November 1992 and December 1992).

Siegel, Bernie. *Love, Medicine and Miracles.* New York: Harper Row, 1986.

————. *Peace, Love and Healing.* New York: Harper Row, 1989.

Tagore, Rabindranath. *Fruit Gathering* LXXIX. 1916. Retrieved May 16, 2003,
    <http://www.iit.edu/-shartan/tagore/fruit.html>

Williams, A. et al.: "Cisplatin Neuropathy with Lhermitte's Sign (letter)" *Journal of Neurology, Neurosurgery, and Psychiatry.* 49:1326 (November 1986). Reprinted in *American Journal of Nursing* (July 1987), p. 52.

Woolhandler, Steffie, and David Himmelstein. "Extreme Risk—The New Corporate Proposition for Physicians." *The New England Journal of Medicine,* vol. 333, no. 25, December 21, 1995.